How to *Love* your *Body* as much as your *Baby*

How to *Love* your *Body* as much as your *Baby*

5 key philosophies to YOUR best ever body!

JEN DUGARD

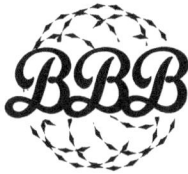

About the Author

Jen Dugard is Australia's leading "mummy trainer". As owner of Body Beyond Baby, Sydney's largest "mum only" exercise company, she heads a team of trainers who are changing the way mums feel about their bodies. Run by mums, for mums, Body Beyond Baby turns tired, self-conscious women who are fed up with their bodies into confident, inspired women who have a great knowledge of health, fitness and nutrition.

Jen trained with the Australian Institute of Fitness, and holds specialist certificates in pre and postnatal exercise. She works closely with women's health physiotherapists, nutritionists, chiropractors and naturopaths to ensure her clients are thoroughly looked after. She is also well-versed in the use of Real Time Ultrasound to assess pelvic floor and transversus abdominis activation.

Body Beyond Baby's success is based on creating communities through exercise, building support networks for mums and challenging them to take time out for themselves.

With one in seven mothers suffering postnatal depression and research suggesting that almost half of women perform incorrect pelvic floor exercises, it's never been more clear that mums need quality advice. Jen is tackling this challenge head-on, and as a result, is helping ease the burden on the Australian healthcare system.

In 2009 Jen produced the postnatal DVD, *Rebuild From The Inside Out*. She delivers regular presentations to mums, has written for the Blackmores Wellbeing Blog, Woolworths Baby and Toddler Club and has featured on the expert panel of newbornbaby.com.au and the Busy Mums' Fitness Club. Jen regularly comments in publications such as *Mother and Baby + Toddler*, *Women's Running* and *The Sun Herald*, and was profiled in a recent video by Isowhey aimed specifically at mums' health and fitness.

CONTACT DETAILS:

Phone: 0402 728 047
Email: jen@jendugard.com
Web/blog: www.jendugard.com

Acknowledgements

The journey to the creation of my first (but not last) book is an ongoing adventure, I feel truly thankful to be able to spend my days doing what I love, helping people and making a difference.

A big thank you goes out to the following people;

Ben; for your unconditional love and support. For being an amazing father and for holding the fort. You allow me to chase my dreams and be everything I want to be, for that I am truly thankful.

My children, Marley and India; without you I would not be doing what I do today. Becoming a mother changed my world and I know my personal experiences have been invaluable in writing this book, doing what I do and the reason I get out of bed in the morning.

Mum and Dad; who always gave me the freedom and confidence to follow my dreams (to the other side of the world).

Sarah; my sister and my friend.

Michaela; for being my sounding board, voice of reason, unwavering support and best friend ever.

Sharon, Amy, Pam and Sally; your energy and support is amazing.

Michaela, Sharon, Amy, Pam and Sally; your energy and support is amazing.

Glen, and Dan; for sparking the journey of a lifetime – and it's only the beginning.

Andrew, Kylie, Mark and Ian; for the inside knowledge on getting every bit right.

Anneka for keeping me on track, being my sounding board, friend and GSD.

The wonderful women who contributed to this book and those I spend my days with, your individual journey's and motivation inspires me, your support and friendship humbles me.

And to everyone reading this book for caring about YOU, for taking the steps to be the best you can be for yourself, your baby and those around you AND for spreading my word that little bit further.

Contents

Nurture from the Inside out 133

Preparation and consistency are key 169

Teach your Children Great Habits................ 185

Introduction

I have written this book for all mothers. In short, I am a mother on a mission – a mission to redefine what it means to be a mother today. I will help you become the best mother you can be, and help you to discover exactly what that means for you.

Through this book, I will help you to figure out what YOUR best body means to you. I will give you the strength, motivation and courage to strive to achieve all of your health and fitness goals, even the ones you may have given up on because of motherhood.

I am bringing back communities through exercise. I am building support networks for mums and providing the means by which they can be the best women and mothers they have ever been.

I am a mother of two beautiful, young children, and I can honestly say that without them I wouldn't be doing what I do today. Yes, I was a personal trainer before my son was born in 2008, but I was working in a large gym chain servicing the masses. It was three months after the birth of my son that I realised what I wanted to do. I was on a journey of my own to navigate my new life, stay healthy, and get back into shape. I was lucky that I had the information and tools necessary to get where I wanted to be, but what I realised was that many of the mums around me really didn't know where to start. They were tired, emotionally and physically drained, often lacked support to find the time for exercise. If they did manage to find the time, they often didn't use it in the most effective way. It was against this background that I decided to launch my business.

I speak to mothers everyday who feel guilty about wanting to do something for themselves. They feel guilty about the thought of leaving their babies to exercise or to make time for themselves. They figure their body can never be what is once was, so what's the point in slogging it out in a gym? They have backache, shoulder pain and mummy tummies, their pelvic floor is shot and an orgasm is a thing of the past. I speak to women who shy away from cameras and miss the opportunity to create lasting memories with their babies because they hate to see themselves in photographs, they struggle to get dressed each day and hide their bodies under baggy clothing.

I understand there is great pressure on women to look a certain way. The media is full of images of celebrities who

How to love your body as much as your baby

seem to bounce back into shape just weeks after giving birth. I am certainly not here to add to any of that pressure. What I am here to do is to show you how to be the very best version of yourself. This is a different picture for each of us, and there is no judgment or expectation, just the goals you set for yourself.

I grew up in the UK and have a background in competitive gymnastics, competing at a national level before moving into gymnastics coaching. I moved to Australia at the age of 18 and spent the first five years carving a career for myself in the film industry. In the years between stopping competitive gymnastics and finding my way back into a gym, my weight increased. My diet was terrible, I was a vegetarian who ate very few vegetables but lots of refined carbohydrates, and I wasn't doing much exercise. It was a fun five years but not a particularly healthy five, working long hours, drinking and partying (not that unusual for a female in her early 20s, I guess). I was drawn back to the health and fitness world when I started training with a personal trainer. This is when my fitness journey really began.

After a while of just increasing exercise, I also started making changes to my diet. At first I was just trying to be healthier but my new healthier attitude towards food started to become more and more restrictive. My diet consisted of salads and vegetarian proteins (soy, tofu, etc.) and not much else. My weight dropped to an unhealthy level. At the time, I thought I loved being tiny, but, thinking about food, my next meal and what I could and couldn't eat started to take over my thinking. I would study the back of food packaging to see which brand had even one or two calories less than the next. Sometimes I would fall off the wagon and binge. It's a little scary admitting all of this in my book but I think that it is important for you to know my past and my experiences and understand that I can relate to the challenges that many women experience. There were times in my life when I made myself vomit after eating too much. Even now, I occasionally have thoughts of doing the same but I have never actually been back there. I now know that if I exercise and eat right I can be in control in a much better way.

I definitely attribute getting married and having a baby to gaining a greater respect for my body, what it is capable of, and how I should treat it. I am not saying that having a child is a cure-all for unhealthy habits (and in fact, for some women, it has the opposite effect) but for me I felt that I had a license to gain weight in a totally acceptable way, along with a drive to stay healthy for my unborn baby. Following the birth, I then had the opportunity to reset my metabolism and lose the weight I had gained during pregnancy in a healthy way. The process allowed me to find a weight and a body fat percentage that was healthy and right for me.

I have documented both of my post baby journeys on my blog (www.jendugard.com) so you can read further if you wish to. I have been through the ups of an 'easier' baby and the downs of postnatal depression. My first child, my son, was a dream baby. He ate and slept and did everything he was supposed to do, in the order that he was supposed to do it. Then two years later, we welcomed our daughter, India, and what followed was 18 months of sleepless nights and a constantly crying baby. I found myself wanting to apologise to the mothers in my original mothers' group, as I had never truly understood what it meant to endure ongoing sleepless nights.

My own post baby journey has shown me some very interesting things. For example, one year after the birth of my daughter, in 2011, I reached the same body fat percentage as I'd had in 2007 but in 2011 I was six kilograms heavier. This is a great example of why you shouldn't trust the scales. How could I possibly weigh six kilograms more and not be fatter? We will touch upon this later, but this was a clear sign that I had my exercise routine and nutrition on track.

My headspace around this time was still not one hundred percent. I spent the first six weeks of India's life in tears. I was still running the organisational side of my business and struggling to figure out how to bathe a two-year old while trying to look after a newborn. Thankfully, my mum came from the UK to help and stayed for 12 months. However, when she left a year later, it was like being transported back to that six-week mark. I was once again all alone, struggling to figure out life with two children. I remember one day, a week after my mother had left, being so frustrated that I put both my children into the bath fully clothed. I eventually found my way through, and things are better now. I still have my ups and downs, but I ask for support when I need it, and I really use my exercise to keep me on track.

My business, Body Beyond Baby, was born in 2008, when my son, Marley, was three-months old. What began as five or six mums and their babies running around the park has since grown, in 2013, to 15 group exercise sessions a week with onsite childcare. Each of the trainers who work with me, were originally members of our mums' groups. Each of these women has changed their life, benefited from their Body Beyond Baby journey and now want to share those experiences with other women.

I have developed close working relationships with other health and fitness professionals, physiotherapists, naturopaths, nutritionists and chiropractors, etc., and spend much of my time learning and refining the techniques which we use on a daily basis to ensure that we are providing the most effective and supportive environment we can for both mothers and their babies.

After working with hundreds of mums, I have discovered five key factors that get in the way of women being individuals as well as mothers. It is these five factors that cause women to lose a sense of who they really are, and prevents them from looking and feeling amazing.

The first factor is a lack of time. They go from taking care of themselves while pregnant, to being so wrapped up with their new baby that they forget to take any time out to rest and rejuvenate. For some mums this can go on for years. They don't realise that in order to be the best mother they can be for their child, they really need to make sure they are well looked after and give themselves the opportunity to be happy first.

How to love your body as much as your baby

The second factor is not knowing where to start to get their bodies back in shape. Many women don't take the time to understand exactly what is happening on the inside from a health and fitness perspective, or what exercises are safe to do soon after childbirth. Add to this not knowing what exercise will be the most effective and sustainable, and many mums are ready to give up before they have even started!

The third factor is confusion about food, what is the best thing to eat and when. Sometimes this is as simple as remembering to eat.

Factor four is the difficulty of making exercise and healthy eating part of a daily routine, particularly if they have little support or help.

The fifth factor is the guilt and stress surrounding the desire to the right thing for their child.

With all this in mind, I have identified five key concepts that you need to know in order to be the best mother you can be and achieve YOUR best ever body both inside and out.

It's not about conforming to the media's idea of a perfect body but about deciding what YOUR best body looks like, how YOU want to feel and who YOU want to be.

The five key concepts are:

Happy Mummy, Happy Baby

I encourage all mums to be a little selfish. Being a mum can be all consuming. From the moment you wake, you are constantly thinking about your child. No matter what kind of mum you are or what kind of parenting techniques you use, we all have one thing in common – we want to be the best possible parent. Around one in seven mothers experience postnatal depression and taking some time out for yourself is so vital to creating a happy mummy, happy baby partnership.

Rebuild from the Inside Out

I believe the absolute key to getting your body back is to understand what is happening on the inside so that you can lay the foundations for YOUR best ever body. After you have laid great foundations, I can then show you how to safely and effectively build the fancy house and create a body and life-style that will last forever.

Nurture from the Inside Out

This is where I relieve the confusion around diet and give simple, effective and easy-to-implement strategies around food and nutrition that will last you a lifetime.

Preparation and Consistency

I know that without being prepared and without being consistent, all the other information is useless. I will show you

How to love your body as much as your baby

techniques to ensure that you prepare for, and keep on track with, achieving YOUR best ever body.

Teach your Children Great Habits

Creating great habits will not only affect you but also your children, and will set them on the right track for life.

When you make the decision to really educate yourself on healthy eating and take the time to exercise, it filters through to the rest of the family. As mothers we often have the huge responsibility of teaching our children how to eat and how often to move. I will help you to get this right.

This book will take you through all you need to know to get started, and share with you the real life experiences of mums I have worked with. The women who have chosen to share their stories in this book have done so with the aim of helping other mothers realise that they are not alone.

The end result will be you developing YOUR own unique plan to achieve YOUR best ever body.

I have also spent time talking with other health professionals and experts who all share a special interest in the wellbeing of mums. They will offer you their expert tips, advice and knowledge.

They say it takes a village to raise a child, so it's no wonder so many women are finding themselves feeling isolated and motherhood to be the hardest and most challenging job they have done in their lives. Through this book, I will show you that it doesn't have to be a lonely journey and that there are groups of women just like you, coming together to discover their own best ever bodies. You can be the strongest, healthiest and sexiest woman you have ever been, even after becoming a mum!

How to use this book

This book is split into sections. Each section contains lots of subheadings so you can easily find your way around, and dip in and out of what you need, when you need. I designed it this way after realising that when you are busy raising a small child, you need to be able to find what you need quickly. This book isn't designed to tell you absolutely everything about health and fitness, but it is designed to be everything you need to know right now.

You may also notice that for a fitness and exercise inspired book there is a serious lack of photographs and picture content. As a trainer I know that it is very difficult to communicate the very best exercise instruction and technique through words on a page or static pictures. I will take you through each exercise in written form but have also created a YouTube channel **(www.youtube.com/JenDugard)** where you can watch me demonstrating all of the exercises included in this book. These videos will provide you with a much better understanding of the techniques, and enable you to exercise more safely and effectively.

I do not believe in a one size fits all solution. So, rather than give you an inflexible program to follow, I will enable you to set your own goals and help you to create a program which can grow and adapt with you, to achieve YOUR best ever body.

I'd also like to invite you to my online Facebook group where you can come and talk to me, ask me questions and share your own journey with others who have also read or who are reading this book. The power is in numbers and the community that we will create.

Enjoy the ride and I look forward to meeting you soon.

Happy Mummy, Happy Baby

I believe it is vital for mothers to find a balance between looking after themselves and looking after their child. In this book
I explore how finding a state of being where you are comfortable with yourself, both mentally and physically, will benefit
your child and create what I have termed a *happy mummy,
happy baby partnership.*

Without a commitment to looking after yourself, and not
just your baby, it will be hard for you to realise what YOUR
best ever body means to you, and to achieve the goals you set
for yourself. You may not even be able to set goals.

Whether you are in the haze of new motherhood, or
have older children and have fallen into the habit of putting
your needs at the bottom of the list, you will benefit from this
book. It will help you to stop, think and decide to take care
of yourself.

I chose to call my book *How to Love your Body as much as your Baby* because I want you to understand that it is okay to want to look and feel fantastic. I want you to feel that you have the right to strive for, and work towards, YOUR best ever body. You don't have to settle for second best now that you are a mum. It's not about conforming to the media's idea of best body, it is about deciding what YOUR best body looks like, how YOU want to feel, what YOU want it to be able to do, and who YOU want to be as well as being a mum. I know that when you look and feel great it can only have a positive impact on your children and family.

Be a little Selfish

Selfish! That's not a word that mums are allowed to comprehend, let alone use. I'd like to, in the nicest possible way, challenge you to be a little bit selfish and to put your own wellbeing at the top of your priority list.

Being a mum can be all consuming. You are constantly thinking about your child and wanting to be the best possible parent. This desire starts in pregnancy, often even before conception, when we devour book after book about how to prepare our bodies for pregnancy and birth, what foods to eat, what exercise to do, what vitamins to take. We read books on the development of our babies as they grow inside us, on the techniques and theories of childbirth, and then we start on parenting techniques. While pregnant, you prepare your meals with care, making sure you include all of the valuable food groups, you rest regularly, you have your personal trainer or Pilates instructor firmly scheduled into your diary, you take regular time out to relax with friends or wind down over a great book and life is great. You are nurturing and loving your baby through your care for your body.

Then your beautiful baby arrives and you continue to devour books, ask questions, worry if they are sleeping too much, eating too little or haven't pooed for two days. The difference is that now your baby is outside of your body you don't have the determination, drive or energy to focus on you any more. But what you forget is that the body that once carried this little baby internally is now the lifeline that carries them externally. Your whole life is centred around them, and will continue to be for the next 18-20 (or more!!) years in one way or another. You are the foundation by which they will learn life, be nurtured and grow into this world.

> ## Your health and wellbeing has never been so important

Many new mothers I meet are doing the most physical job they have EVER done, in the most physically de-conditioned state they have ever been in. Add to this sleep deprivation, being constantly 'on call' and not managing to eat before lunchtime, and you have a recipe for disaster.

I truly believe there has never been a better time to teach mothers how important it is to look after themselves, to be fit, healthy and strong for the benefit of their children. I work with mums on a daily basis and I know that when they change their outlook and attitude to focus on living a healthier and more active life, their children benefit hugely.

> # Energy creates energy

You, Mum, are the building block of your family. Your influence is second to none, and by remembering to fit your own oxygen mask first, your whole family will reap the rewards.

Take a little Time Out

When you are in the baby bubble and your world is a blur of naps and feeding and you haven't even managed to get in the shower for two days it is hard to see how you can actually do something for yourself.

This doesn't stop when your baby gets older, there's always the washing and the cleaning, the drop-offs and the activities, going back to work and really, just LIFE! Life is a challenge. For many of you I know it is busy, it doesn't stop, there is no end to the list of the things that need doing and no sooner have you crossed one thing off then five others have been added to the bottom but this is where it has to stop.

Right here, right now. You are the backbone of your family, you are the glue that holds it all together and you need a break. You need to recharge your batteries and you need to MAKE time for yourself.

Make time for yourself

I can't stress how important it is to make time for yourself. You need to know that on a daily basis you are doing something for you. It doesn't have to be a big thing to begin with; a shower might be the right thing to get started with – put your baby in a safe place and take the shower. Not a 30 second shower but one that allows you to wash it all away, that gives you time to really feel the water splashing over you, that reminds you that you are important and you need some attention too. As time progresses and when you feel ready, begin to commit to some other specific and planned times that are all about you. That are scheduled into your day just like your child's activities or nap times are scheduled into your day. There is nothing selfish about making sure that you are in the right mental, emotional and physical state to look after your child.

In today's society, many of us are raising children without extended family around us. In my experience, this lack of support contributes greatly towards the incidence of postnatal depression.

My Story

Prior to having a baby I had experienced periods of feeling depressed and so when I had my first child I actually expected to experience some symptoms of postnatal depression (PND) but I just seemed to cruise on through. Marley was a relatively easy baby and he slept. I almost wasn't sure what all the fuss was about when other people told me how hard it was being a mum. I started my business, Body Beyond Baby, when Marley was three months old, in my quest to add something else to my life. I continued to cruise on through, build my business and enjoy my boy.

The second time around, things were different. I was already entering into pregnancy and birth with a lot fewer reserves – small children don't let you rest like you did in your first pregnancy and it's certainly not all about you anymore. I was running my growing business and although I had organised another trainer to fill in the delivery of sessions for six months, there was no stopping in terms of the behind the scenes running of my business.

When India arrived exactly two years (to the day!) later I was so excited to have a little girl in my life, but my experience with her was completely different to what I had experienced with Marley. From day one she didn't sleep, she was called a 'highly and easily stimulated baby' who just seemed to cry and cry and cry. I got to the point where to try to calm her down I sat in a darkened room for three days, only coming out when she was sleeping. This was doable for three days but not a way

How to love your body as much as your baby

to live life. I remember dragging myself out to one of those mothers' group meetings at an early childhood centre and saying I had absolutely no idea how I was supposed to look after both of them. I spent the first six weeks of India's life in tears.

I was never diagnosed with PND but I know that's what I was experiencing. The seemingly endless nights of broken sleep lasted for 18 months. I remember one, middle of the night experience where I literally couldn't take it anymore and almost threw India at my husband; it was then that I knew I needed help. I was extremely blessed that at the six-week mark my mum came to Sydney from England for a year-long stay. This pulled me out of my hole and relieved a lot of pressure because I was no longer doing the day-to-day alone. Mum was amazing with my children and she enabled me to take some much needed time out.

Throughout this whole experience, my commitment to my own exercise routine was one of the things that kept my head above water.

There are still days when I don't want to get off the couch and I don't want to work and exercise feels too hard, but I am lucky to be surrounded by a fantastic. I surround myself with inspiring and motivated people, which in turn motivates me. This is the aim of the group training component of Body Beyond Baby and our online networks. We are creating communities who come together through health and fitness; they inspire, motivate and support each other. Many of the mums I work with form friendships that carry into their lives outside of training, and it's amazing to be part of such a wonderful group of women who have the courage to make sure they are helping themselves. I encourage you to find some exercise you love and to do the same.

Postnatal Depression (PND)

Around one in seven new mothers experiences postnatal depression (PND). Research out of the UK suggests that over 50 percent of mums with PND are suffering in silence. Anxiety is even more common, and both anxiety and depression can also occur during pregnancy. Keeping active is a good way to help prevent or manage mild to moderate depression and anxiety.

> # Women supporting women

There are many views as to how exercise helps people with depression. On a simple level, exercise can distract you from daily worries.

On a more scientific level, exercise is known to increase levels of neurotransmitters (chemical messengers in the brain) that have been found to be in short supply when you are depressed. Exercise also increases endorphins, which are chemicals in the brain that have mood-lifting qualities.

A number of studies have found that exercise helps depression. Jogging, weightlifting, walking, stationary cycling

How to love your body as much as your baby

and resistance training have all been found to be helpful in preventing or treating mild to moderate depression.

If you are suffering from PND there may be a number of barriers stopping you from exercising regularly. Finding the motivation to get started can be very difficult and that is where the importance of an exercise community comes in. I firmly believe in the power of a group, communities of women that come together to support each other through tough and challenging times. There are many views as to how exercise can help you overcome or manage PND. Exercise may block negative thoughts or distract people from their worries. If that person is exercising within a group it increases their social contact.

Exercise may also change levels of chemicals in the brain, such as serotonin, endorphins and stress hormones. A number of studies have found that exercise helps depression. One study has reported that total energy expenditure is a key factor in the remission of depression. Leading authors recommend that individuals should be encouraged to do at least 30 minutes of moderate intensity exercise on most, if not all, days of the week.

Keeping active can not only help you to stay physically fit but mentally fit too. Research shows that keeping active can:

- help lift mood
- help get a good nights sleep (if your baby cooperates too!)
- increase energy levels

- help block negative thoughts and/or distract people from daily worries
- help people feel less alone if they exercise or socialise with others
- increase wellbeing

Create a community around you

Through my own personal experience and having worked with a number of mums suffering from PND, it is apparent that creating a community around you at this time can be hugely beneficial in overcoming your negative feelings. It may take a little effort to begin with but realising that you don't have to do this alone can be a huge relief. You need to surround yourself with healthy and positive people, mothers who can relate to what you are going through and who can offer you encouragement, support and a sense of wellbeing.

Through my business, Body Beyond Baby, I launched a community initiative called The Bluebird Community. Under this initiative, we partner with other businesses (who offer sponsorship) and other health professionals (who refer women suffering from PND), and offer women with PND the opportunity to exercise with us for a period of time at no cost. We have had some fantastic results and really see the benefit for mums with PND to be able to easily access exercise, without having to worry about where to go or the financial cost.

If you think you may be suffering from PND I suggest you seek out a community, either face-to-face or online. There are fantastic charities like *beyondblue*, and the Gidget Foundation which are there to help. You can also join our online Facebook page where you will experience the support and encouragement of other mums going through similar experiences.

Ask for help

You have no idea how many mums I meet who just don't ask for help. I understand that many of you are living far away from family, have partners who work long hours, or you may just not know anyone else with children, but I urge you to seek out a few key people who are happy to help. You would be surprised at how many people would love to spend time with your child, to give you a little break, if you asked. Before we moved to our current home we lived in a beautiful block of apartments in Randwick. When we moved in I was pregnant with my son and instantly we were welcomed. We walked into one of those rare blocks in Sydney where everyone knew each other and cared about each other. Almost all of the neighbours had keys to at least one other person's home and we could knock on any door and ask for a cup of milk or an onion when we had run out. Helping hands were made available to me by some of the most unlikely people in that apartment block, but that was only after I decided to ask for help.

Asking for help, or allowing people to help you, can be challenging. We all feel like we know our baby best, and that they need us and might be upset without us. It is true, your child may take a little extra time to settle with somebody else, but the value to you when you are completely exhausted will be worth it. This doesn't have to be a big change, take baby steps and go at your own pace. First try 15 minutes to take a shower, then a 30minute walk – keep your phone on you and do what works for you to make sure it's not adding stress. The more time your baby spends with somebody else the more they will get to know each other and the less time that settling will take.

I know many mums who don't even leave their child with their partner. I've witnessed scenarios where dad has been trying to do something for their child, only to be told he is doing it wrong or that she prefers it done another way. I've been there myself, where you believe your way is the only way, and the quickest way to stop your child from being upset. Again, in this instance you may be able to settle your child more quickly, but by taking away your partner's opportunity to learn and get to know your baby, his baby, you are taking away your opportunity for some much needed you time. Your baby and your partner need to get to know each other too. One of the best things I learned to do when my babies were really little was to just walk away and leave them to it. There were times, of course, where I didn't, where I jumped in and took over with the 'he likes it like this', and 'you don't do it like that'. However, there were other times where I did leave

How to love your body as much as your baby

them to it, and it took all my willpower not to intervene, but I can't tell you how awesome it is now for my children to have such a hands on dad. Half the time I swear he does a better parenting job than I do.

> # Let your child and partner learn about each other

One really important thing to remember is that nine times out of ten your child's father and/or your partner really wants to help. So don't discourage help by being too particular. No one likes to be criticised for their efforts. Give your partner a chance, without judgment or criticism, to figure out the best way for themselves and your baby – it might not be your way, but that doesn't mean it's wrong.

Introducing Dr Nicole Highet

Dr Nicole Highet is a leading Australian expert in perinatal mental health. She completed a doctorate in the perinatal area and has worked for the last 12 years at *beyondblue* which is a charity aimed at achieving an Australian community that understands depression and anxiety and empowers individuals to seek help. Nicole also co-chaired the development of the Perinatal Clinical Practice Guidelines, endorsed by the National Health and Medical Research Council in May 2011, and expanded this to include online accredited training programs and education resources for health professionals, women and their families.

Nicole's current focus is working to establish a new, independent *Centre of Perinatal Excellence* for Australia. The Centre will build on the work of *beyondblue* to equip health professionals with the knowledge and tools to undertake screening for postnatal depression, and to provide effective treatments. In addition, the Centre will ensure women and their families have timely access to high quality campaigns, information and services.

Nicole's top 5 expert tips to help to prevent PND

1. **Educate yourself** – before you have a baby, read as much as you can about PND, understand the symptoms and know what to look out for.

2. **Be aware of your expectations of being a mother** – think about your expectations of motherhood and try to be realistic.

3. **Prepare yourself** for the challenges of motherhood and acknowledge that there will be good days and bad days.

4. **Eat well** – make sure you nurture your body during pregnancy to keep you and your baby healthy.

5. **Make sure you exercise** during your pregnancy (unless instructed otherwise by your doctor) and after the baby is born. Being healthy, fit and strong will ensure that you are in the best possible physical condition to deal with the challenges of motherhood.
It can also prevent mental health problems occurring in some women.

More from Nicole

Depression and anxiety are very common mental health problems. Statistics show that women most often experience depression and anxiety around pregnancy and childbirth. Anxiety and depression can often occur at the same time – in fact in up to 50 percent of cases. It is important for women to be aware of the symptoms and early warning signs of anxiety and depression so that they can seek help if necessary.

There are a number of factors that place people at particular risk of suffering from anxiety and depression. One of the key risk factors is having a history of depression or anxiety. If you have experienced depression or anxiety before pregnancy, you need to be especially vigilant to look out for warning signs and be sure to ask for help if you see the signs.

Another major risk factor is a lack of social support. For women without an established support network, motherhood can be a very isolating experience. For those women who do not have families or other support networks readily available, it is important to build networks, for example through joining a mothers' group.

Happy Mummy, Happy Baby

Common warning signs of depression and/or anxiety:

- You feel like you are struggling to cope to get through the day
- You are not enjoying life or the things that you used to get pleasure from
- You are not enjoying your baby
- You are feeling the desire to isolate yourself
- You feel constantly anxious or worried that something terrible is going to happen to your baby

What you can look out for in others:

It is important to look out for signs of anxiety and depression in women around you. If you notice a change in someone's disposition or they seem to be less socially connected, or less outgoing this can be an indicator of anxiety or depression. Women can be very good at pretending that everything is great, so be aware of more subtle signs too.

The media often creates unrealistic expectations of motherhood and it is these expectations that can cause disappointment and feelings of failure. In reality, there will be many difficult days and it's important to be realistic and honest about that, and ask for support if you are struggling. Within every mothers' group, there is likely to be at least one mum who will experience anxiety or depression and so it is important to look out for signs and offer support if you suspect someone is struggling.

It's important to remember that suffering from depression or anxiety is not a reflection of you as a person, or as a mother. Everyone has different experiences; some people have more difficult births, difficult pregnancies, difficulty getting pregnant or a more difficult baby. There is no point in comparing yourself to others; the important thing is to recognise if you need help and to be supportive to those who are struggling.

It is really important to feel good about yourself after having a baby. Mental health issues are often closely related to self-esteem. How you feel about yourself physically, in terms of strength and fitness, and how you feel about yourself when you look in the mirror, can have a significant impact on your mental health. With this in mind, it is important to work towards getting yourself into a physical state that you are comfortable with, and that prepares you for the challenges of motherhood.

"Happy Mummy, Happy Baby" is an important philosophy. If you feel good about yourself, this will affect all aspects of your life, your relationships, your willingness and interest in socialising and being active, and all this will in turn improve the quality of your interaction with your baby.

Real Mums

Elizabeth, mum to Jack(6), Alex(3) and currently pregnant with number three

It might sound like an odd thing to say, especially to someone who's currently going through PND, but for me, getting PND ended up being an absolute blessing. I suffered from PND after the births of both my boys. The first time I put it down to sleep deprivation and the belief that parenting was just hard and not necessarily enjoyable and so I just muddled through. How untrue, and what a massive waste of Jack's first year. After the arrival of my second child, Alex, it took no time before I was back at rock bottom; constant tears, the inability to think and make decisions, let alone being able to look after two kids. What I did this time though, massively improved my mood, energy (despite sleep deprivation) and my ability to enjoy parenting. I decided I needed to do whatever it took to feel better so I could see what all the fuss of parenting was about. I started to eat more healthily and more regularly, sought my doctor's advice and went on medication. I also began exercising with Jen at Body Beyond Baby as soon as I'd had my 6-week check-up. This turned out to be the key turning point.

Training with an exercise professional who specialises in postnatal exercise, teaching the importance of safely rebuilding strength from the inside out, made all the difference. Before long I felt stronger and fitter than I had in years. The nannies took

How to love your body as much as your baby

care of the kids while I got fresh air, sunshine (also a brilliant cure for depression), increased strength, social activity with other mums, and a hit of endorphins.

Despite only being able to commit to one session a week, this turned out to be enough to spur me on and provide me with tips for doing more exercise on my own throughout the rest of the week. Now, almost two years on, I still hold exercise as *the* most important factor for boosting my mood, my ability to cope and my ability to think clearly. I don't live in Sydney anymore, so can't train with Jen, but if you do, I couldn't recommend training with Jen more highly. She is so passionate about what she does, she practices what she preaches, is genuinely interested in each of the mums and I am still in contact with her despite being interstate.

As someone who's had quite an ongoing history of depression, especially in times of big changes (e.g. moving house/country, changing jobs and having a baby) I can say with experience that good regular exercise (not just walking) doesn't get the emphasis it should. Talking to a psychologist or medication alone isn't enough. I now know that exercise and nutrition are absolutely vital in truly getting your life turned around for the long term.

Virginia, Mum to Jake(8), Jesse(6) and Lili(3)

Coming from a strong blood line of women, depression was never something I thought would happen to me. I grew up a happy, confident kid in Perth, always had lots of friends, did well at school and university, travelled the world, enjoyed a successful corporate career for many years and always worked hard to achieve my goals. I was invincible (or so I thought), three kids...piece of cake!

For me, the warning signs started when my third baby, Lili, was just a few months old, although looking back I'm fairly certain I had the same signs with my second. She, like the boys, was delivered by caesarean and I was over the moon that we finally had the coveted baby girl of whom I had dreamed. Not long after the hormones settled down, reality kicked in and I was faced with having to juggle a newborn baby, a very strong-willed three-year old (not at all happy with his new sibling) and a five-year old just starting primary school. I'd wake up feeling utterly exhausted, having been up all night breastfeeding or settling...then having to pick myself up and pretend everything was normal – packing lunches, getting three kids ready for the day and the dreaded morning drop-offs in the pouring rain with baby on one hip, umbrella and school bags in one hand, little hands in the other. One morning it was raining so heavily, I slipped and fell into the gutter (luckily didn't drop the baby). Tears running down my face, completely drenched and not knowing which way was up or down, I managed to get up and get the boys to school

How to love your body as much as your baby

and kindy safely (albeit saturated) and I spent the next hour or so howling in my car. What happened to my life? What have I become?

Next came feelings of being completely overwhelmed, a failure, alone and resentful, anxiety attacks, frequent crying and feeling completely unsatisfied in life. My coping mechanisms had hit rock bottom. With my own family and close friends in Perth, I didn't have a strong support network to begin with and started to withdraw from social circles because it was just all too hard. I was cranky with my husband, short fused with the kids and behaving like a complete maniac and I didn't have the power to stop. I thought to myself, 'Pick yourself up Virginia, plenty of women have walked in your shoes, you can do this,' but I soon realised these feelings weren't going away and something had to change.

My obstetrician suggested I talk to someone, which I did, and was shortly thereafter diagnosed with PND. I was gutted and relieved at the same time, but at least I knew what was going on in my head. After a few sessions I soon realised that, like most women, I was (and still am) constantly placing unrealistic pressure on myself to do everything, be everything to everyone, all the while being polite with a smile on my face! I had to start making some changes in my life and start learning to be kinder to myself. So I started scheduling in some me time – diarising events with friends and date nights with the husband, got myself a cleaner and started exercising again.

Happy Mummy, Happy Baby

While many of my friends were falling prey to PND and the medication route, for me, exercise was the first and natural choice, as I'd always been heavily into sports growing up and never had the time to get back into it with kids. I am so grateful I stumbled across Jen Dugard's Body Beyond Baby through a friend because it has been my saving grace, literally. Not only is it cheaper than therapy (much!), but it also alleviated the stress of trying to find a babysitter via Body Beyond Baby's nanny service. I now exercise daily (three weekly sessions with Body Beyond Baby) and I am pleased to say I am not only feeling the best I've felt in years, but I've also regained my self confidence and wake up in the morning with a smile on my face and a spring in my step. There is nothing quite like the feeling of a natural endorphin high, and I am proud to say my PND days are behind me. Rocking a pair of killer heels and skinny jeans has never been more enjoyable.

5 Easy To Implement Actions

1. Do one thing EVERY day that is JUST FOR YOU

2. Get out of the house daily – even if it's just for a walk

3. Call a friend and make a date to do some exercise

4. Negotiate time with your partner for them to stay with your baby while you take some Mummy time out – remember, stay comfortable, baby steps to begin with and then increase the time as you feel ready

5. Find your community, join an exercise or walking group, call up your old friends or jump online and start with our supportive Facebook page

Exercise - Part 1

Rebuild from the Inside Out

YOUR Best Ever Body

As a personal trainer I know it is absolutely vital that you are armed with as much knowledge as possible to make achieving YOUR best ever body as pain free, effective and simple as it can be. I like to use the term 'Rebuild from the Inside Out', as I believe this is the absolute key to getting your body back. In fact, if you take the time and energy to really concentrate and rebuild from the inside out, I have no doubt that you can end up fitter and stronger than ever before. Add to this the confidence you gain from looking and feeling great and I know you will also feel sexier than you have ever done in your life.

Your body is amazing

A woman's body is an amazing thing – you have grown and given birth to a baby. You have given love to your body throughout pregnancy and done everything in your power to ensure you did the best possible things for the wellness of your child. Give this body the respect it deserves. You may have war wounds, stretch marks and wobbly bits, but when you learn to love your body and be grateful for the experience it has given you, then you can begin your new journey of discovering YOUR best ever body. I say YOUR because that is what it is – your journey, there is no-one to compare to; only you. In a world where we are surrounded by false images of what it means to be a woman and mother, it is very easy to lose ourselves in comparing our bodies to others. I challenge you to think of only you for a while. What is YOUR best body? What does it look like? What does it feel like? How do you feel now that you are in it? Only you can set the parameters of the body that you want to belong to you. It is then only you who can embark upon the journey to get there. There is no judgment from others about the body you wish to create. The only person you need to satisfy is yourself. I know when you do that, and you are comfortable and confident in the skin you are in, then it will have a positive impact on those around you. They will see that you are happy, healthy and confident and all of that positive energy will rub off on them – it's a win-win for all.

How to love your body as much as your baby

MY Best Ever Body

Set out below, is a description of MY best ever body. Although I am sharing this with you, you need to remember that this is my picture, my journey and, most likely, very different from yours.

My body is strong – I will push myself to take on new challenges and achieve new heights through my health and fitness. As a result, my body looks strong and lean, but still feminine. I like muscles, not too big (maybe bigger than most) but muscles that show I am serious about my fitness routine and healthy eating. I feel confident on the beach in a bikini and sexy in jeans. I have a flat stomach and definition of abdominal muscles (this is actually quite challenging for me but when it happens I know I feel AMAZING; it's just my little physical check-in point). People are surprised when they find out I have a child (more so when they know I have two). I inspire other mothers as to the body they can achieve after having a baby. My body will allow me to play with my children, to really allow me to join in with their games, and teach them new things physically. I can climb a rope or a pole at the park, teach them to cartwheel, and show them what it means to lead a healthy and active life as they grow. I lead by example.

Like I said, this is my account of the body I want to live in – some of it I have achieved and some of it I am still working towards. I challenge you now to really think about the body you would like to create. Start to envisage what it will feel like when you get there, what you will see in the mirror, and how you will feel when you get dressed. What new things will you be able to do? What is important to you and what kind of an example would you like to set for your children?

Next I would like you to write this down, just as I have done, and I would like you to write it as if you are already there. You are already in YOUR best body. You know what it is like and you can feel how you feel. Once you have visualised that body, I can help you get there in the safest and most effective way possible.

Let's start from the inside and everything you need to know about Rebuilding from the Inside Out.

Your Inner Unit

I am sure you know you have a core – they are the bits on the inside, right? Core has been a bit of a buzz word amongst the fitness industry for a number of years now, but I believe there may be a misunderstanding of what your core is, what it does, what it is vital for and how to train it in the most effective way – especially after having a baby.

Your true core, or as I like to call it, Inner Unit, is made up of your transversus abdominis, pelvic floor, diaphragm, and multifidus. In order to make sure that after having a baby you are able to rebuild your body to be the strongest and fittest it has ever been, it is very important to know what is going on, on the inside.

Pelvic Floor

> ## Pelvic floor weakness is not just a by-product of having a baby

Many people think of the pelvic floor as a strip of muscle that goes from the front to back of their pelvis, when in actual fact your pelvic floor is more of a sling or funnel that stretches from both front to back and from side to side of the pelvis. Your pelvic floor is responsible for supporting the organs that sit within your pelvis, your bladder, uterus and rectum. Without a full functioning pelvic floor you can experience various symptoms ranging from slight bladder leakage or urge incontinence, to the more obviously serious such as pro-lapse of the organs (where you can feel or see them coming out). For me, all of these symptoms, no matter how mild, are a warning sign that you need to learn more, and become more aware of your pelvic floor.

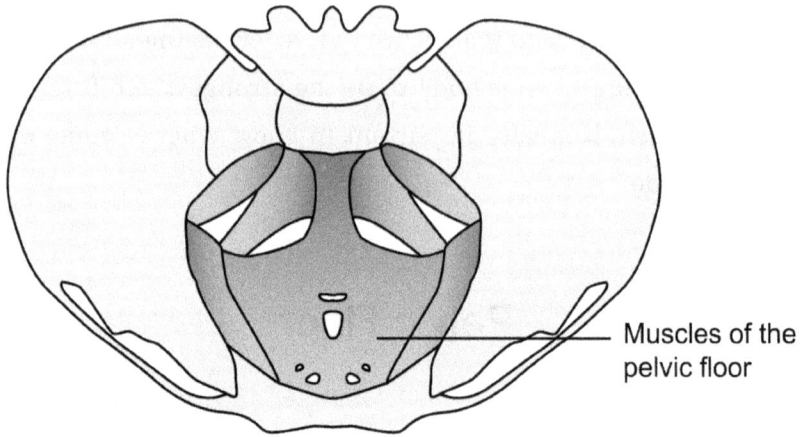

Muscles of the pelvic floor

I speak to many women who are under the impression that urine leakage is just a regular and expected part of being a mother. Their mother and/or grandmother may have mentioned that it happened to them, and therefore they should just accept that it is a by-product of having a baby. I would like to tell you that this isn't so. It is not normal to experience or have to live with any of the following symptoms:

- Bladder or bowel leakage during exercise or at any time
- Urge incontinence (meaning when you need to go you MUST go right that second or risk an accident)
- Any feeling of dragging or heaviness in the pelvic region
- Lack of sensation and/or ability to orgasm

If you are experiencing ANY of the above, then I highly recommend that you seek out the support of an experienced women's health physiotherapist and who can help you to

How to love your body as much as your baby

figure out what is happening with your body. The physio-therapist will help you take your first step towards achieving YOUR best ever body (download the Useful Contacts list from our website for our physiotherapist recommendations).

Pelvic Floor Exercises Unravelled

> An incorrect pelvic floor exercise may do more harm than good

It is documented that only half of the women that read the 'how to do pelvic floor exercises' guide, or are just given a verbal cue of pelvic floor activation, do it correctly. If drawing your pelvic floor up is the correct activation then it only makes sense that an incorrect one would be that of bearing down. I am sure you can imagine that a woman who spends time each day perform-ing many, many incorrect (bearing down) activations is most likely doing her body more damage than good.

I have seen firsthand a client who was on the way to causing a prolapse from doing incorrect activation exercises.

Know how to RELAX your pelvic floor

It is also important that you know how to relax your pelvic floor. Yes, a strong pelvic floor is ideal but it is also just as important to be able to relax too. It has been shown that there is correlation between a hypertonic (overactive) pelvic floor and pelvic girdle pain.

I came across a case of a woman who, since the birth of her first child, had done hundreds of pelvic floor exercises everyday. She had done them, at the traffic lights, feeding her baby, waiting for the kettle to boil. After a straightforward first birth, the result of all those pelvic floor exercises, was the traumatic birth of her second child. The baby wouldn't come out and she ended up with a severe tear. This was put down to her strong pelvic floor and her inability to release those muscles and allow the baby to come out.

I am not saying that doing daily pelvic floor exercises is wrong. I am simply saying that you need to do them well. It is documented that the pelvic floor is an automatic muscle and when working well ('working well' being the key phrase here) there is potentially no need for a daily training program. If you are aware of the correct inner unit activation pattern and have taken the time to rebuild strength and learn how to relax it after having your baby, then ideally your pelvic floor will be automatically trained on a daily basis, without you having to do specific exercises.

For some people a daily retraining program is exactly what they need, but my argument is that by reading this book or working with me you are no longer classified as general public when it comes to knowledge of your pelvic floor. You now know that without proper assessment you could be doing your exercises incorrectly and causing more harm than good. You also know that it is as important to be able to release as well as contract your pelvic floor. With this knowledge, I urge you to seek out the opinion of a qualified and experience physiotherapist who can ensure that you are on track and develop a rehabilitation program that is designed specifically for you (visit our website to download a list of practitioners specialising in women's health and Real Time Ultrasound).

Please visit www.youtube/JenDugard for guidance on how to activate your pelvic floor

Sit-ups will Not give you a Flat Tummy

In my view, sit-ups really should not feature in this section of the book. Sit-ups are one of the most oversubscribed and underperforming exercises that you can waste your (very precious) time doing. They actually play no role in retraining your inner unit. Nevertheless, I have included them here because I know that many people think that to get a flat tummy you need to do lots and lots of sit-ups – how wrong could they be!

Your tummy is made up of four layers of muscle. From the outside you have your rectus abdominus, followed by external obliques, then internal obliques and finally the bottom layer are your transversus abdominis.

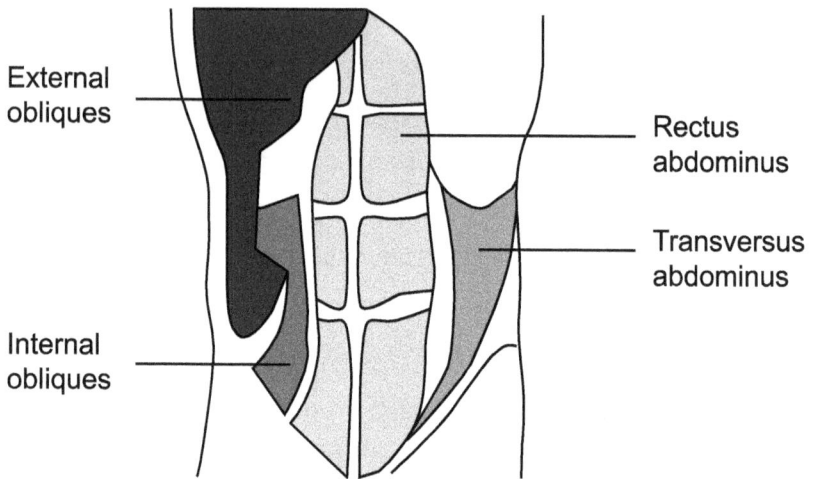

Your rectus abdominus is important for control during flexion and extension of the trunk during daily activities. However, by performing sit-ups you are only training the movement of trunk flexion, they are often far too difficult for people to do well, and as a result can weaken both their transversus abdominis and pelvic floor. Your obliques are responsible for twisting movements.

It is your innermost layer of muscle, your transversus abdominis (TA) that offers that support to your back and acts as a corset around your trunk and in turn, when working well, actually flattens our tummy.

I know that many people, when they think about or start on their mission to regain their flat tummy, perform lots of sit-ups or twisting movements. I can tell you now that these exercises alone will not flatten your mummy tummy. They will not tone your abdominals in the way that you would like. For many of you, if you have any signs of abdominal separation, pelvic floor weakness or weak TA, you may actually be doing yourself damage and could end up making your 'sticky-out' tummy even worse.

Every sit-up you perform creates what we call intra-abdominal pressure and the only place for this pressure to come out is through your pelvic floor if it is weak, or through a weak abdominal wall, putting excess pressure on those places that may already be weakened.

Do you have Abdominal Separation?

You may or may not have heard of abdominal separation and you may or may not have been assessed for separation before you left the hospital after you had your baby. You may be told a separation is normal and will heal automatically. However, anecdotal evidence shows us that is often not the case. Addressing your separation with an individualised exercise program, with or without some compression binding, as soon as possible is crucial to the healing of the separation.

Abdominal separation occurs when the connective tissue, the linea alba, running down the middle of your abdominal wall, that joins all of the abdominal wall muscles starts to tear. The two sides of your rectus abdominus are forced apart due to their inability to stretch anymore and provide any more space for your growing baby. When this happens, the area of connective tissue will then start to give and separate, allowing your baby more room to grow.

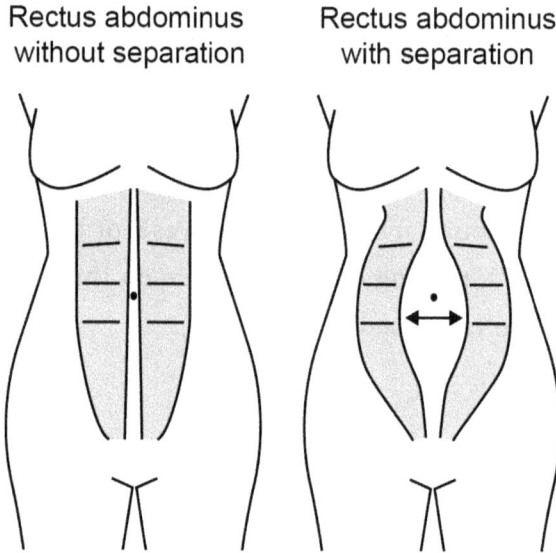

Rectus abdominus without separation

Rectus abdominus with separation

Some women have very little or no abdominal separation at all. It is very normal to have around two fingers of separation, and in more severe cases I have seen four fingers and more. We also now know that it is important to assess both the depth as well as the width of separation – when the separation is deep and you can feel no floor to your abdominals you are at a higher risk of a herniation of your organs through your abdominal wall. I am sure that you can imagine sit-ups performed with a large abdominal separation and weak abdominal wall can not be doing you any good (and may in fact make your tummy stick out even further).

How to check for abdominal separation

Here is a step-by-step guide to checking yourself for abdominal separation. You can also visit my YouTube channel for my how-to guide to check your own abdominal separation.

- Lie down on your back, knees bent and feet flat on the floor, shoulders relaxed
- Place two fingers just below your belly button
- Slowly roll your shoulders off the floor into a mini sit-up (avoid over tensing your tummy muscles)
- Using your two fingers feel the gap between your two rectus abdominus
- Measure the gap below your belly button then repeat above and up to your rib cage

You should also feel for the floor in your separation, as depth is as important as width. If there is no floor or it is very spongy and deep (sometimes you can feel right down to your organs), it is more severe than if you can feel separation but there is no depth at all i.e. your abdominal wall is right there, strong despite any gap.

What is normal and what does it mean?

Firstly, having a gap after being pregnant is very normal, and given we are all different and all on our own journey, you shouldn't feel like the depth or width or your separation is any better or worse than others – just some of you may have less or more work to do than others at this point.

A two finger gap

In my experience a gap of two fingers is quite common – I find many new mums are starting at this point and with the correct rebuilding exercises this gap will completely close.

Less than two fingers

Some of you will discover you have less than two fingers separation or none at all, and this is great. However, in the early stages of your rebuilding process my recommendation would be to treat yourself as if you did have a gap and to make sure you perfect our TA activation and breathing exercise, as you still need to ensure that your inner unit is working properly and effectively to rebuild to be the strongest you have ever been.

It is often within this category that I see mums who have had no separation launch back in to sit-ups and twisting movements because there is no obvious reason not to. But by doing this, they have neglected to rebuild from the inside out and often end up with injuries and backaches down the track. If you fall into this category, know that rebuilding from the inside out is still absolutely vital on your journey to YOUR best ever body.

More than two fingers

If you have a gap more than two fingers wide and/or it is very deep, you fall into the category of those who have a little more work to do. Remember, by having this information you are now equipped with the best possible knowledge to rebuild and discover YOUR best body yet. There are not many times in life when we allow ourselves to slow down and really take a look from the inside, to work in the best possible way to ensure we are stronger and fitter than we have ever been in the past. In my opinion, there is a huge number of the general population who would benefit greatly from this knowledge, and from taking the time to ensure that their inner unit is working properly and effectively. Many of the corporate professionals who are sitting day after day at a desk with poor posture; pelvic tilts (which is shown to inhibit pelvic floor activation), relaxed and poorly activating transverse abdominals (which are doing nothing to protect their backs) or hunched shoulders (which is a sign of weak rhomboids and a tight chest) could very much benefit from the knowledge that you now have. They may not have abdominal separation, but they certainly don't have an effectively working inner unit, and are likely to be suffering from backache and poor posture for a very long time.

If you do have a larger separation it is extremely important that you take the right steps to ensure you fix it. By doing incorrect exercises at this stage, with a gap and a weakened abdominal wall, you could easily end up making it worse and potentially causing a herniation.

Correcting abdominal separation

When faced with a mummy tummy and abdominal separation it is easy to just do what you think you should do. But, as we have touched on earlier, sit-ups at this stage of the game could be one of the most damaging exercises you could choose. If you have already started doing them, don't worry too much; just stop now that you have more knowledge and information to work with. You don't know what you don't know, and be aware of what advice you take when it comes to correcting your separation. If you are ever in a situation where you are told to 'do a few sit-ups and in time it will go away', know now that this isn't the case and that performing incorrect exercises at this time could lead to further damage.

A great analogy I like to use is that you wouldn't go and see an eye specialist in hope that they could fix your knee. You may be seated in front of the best ophthalmologist in the world, but if you think they are going to be able to offer you the best possible care for your knee you would be mistaken. Most people know this; it's plain common sense, but I see many people trusting their bodies with others who know nothing about, and have no experience with, the care that they need.

When choosing to work with someone for your postnatal care, look at their specialities, find out what type of person they work with or whether they have been through something from a personal point of view. If it is a personal trainer you are in search of, I believe that a really great PT will know what they don't know – if your trainer has referred you on to another trainer because they know you could get better care with someone else, you know you are in good hands. Or if they recommend you see another health professional so that they can work with them within a network of care, and they communicate with these other health professionals, again, you know you are on the right track. I believe it is vital to know what I don't know. I am not a physiotherapist or gynaecologist. I am well versed in many of the signs to look out for when assessing abdominal separation, pelvic floor or TA activation, but there is only so much I can do through touch and feel. If I want to truly know what is happening with someone on the inside, then I need to call upon my network of trusted health professionals to work with me and manage each case on an individual basis.

How do you fix separation?

We now know that sit-ups won't fix your separation. I feel the need to say that over and over and over again because sometimes people keep doing what they know and hope for the best. I will go as far as to say that if you never, ever, did another sit-up in your life it would not be a bad thing. You can still achieve a flat and toned abdominal wall and, more than likely, end up much, much stronger through your inner unit, by performing a variety of other core strengthening exercises than if you concentrate on sit-ups alone.

The first thing you need to know about fixing separation and building TA strength is exactly the title of this chapter – you need to Rebuild from the Inside Out. Going back to what we said before, may people think that to achieve a toned or flat tummy you need to do lots of sit-up and twisting movements. We know from earlier in this chapter that sit-ups work your rectus abdominus (responsible for flexion of the trunk) and twisting movements work your obliques. So your rectus abdominus runs from top to bottom, your obliques run on a diagonal and your TA runs horizontally and connects from your ribs right around the back. It connects to your linea alba, which is the connective tissue between your rectus abdominus, the bit that can separate, causing your gap.

If we think about this further, it makes sense that when you work your rectus abdominus, you could add intra-abdominal pressure to a weak abdominal wall and potentially push your rectus further apart. When you overwork your obliques they can increase force to the linea alba and make your separation worse. I refer to building strength in your rectus and obliques as building the fancy house; you may do all of the exercises that I don't recommend and your tummy could, for a while, look great. But bit by bit you start to get a niggle through your back, hip pain or a knee injury, and with further research it is discovered that your TA is not working in the most effective way. You skipped the laying of the foundations and got carried away building the fancy house. We all know the story of the three little pigs and the pig who rushed to build a pretty house, but it was blown over all too easily when the big bad wolf came along. I can't stress highly enough the importance or benefits of rebuilding from the inside out.

A great example of this is that I recently had a client who underwent surgery to fix her separation – unfortunately there are certain cases that we cannot fix through exercise alone. I went with her to some of her pre-op and post-op appointments to meet the surgeon, learn more about the procedure and what was advised for after the operation. One of the key things he said that really stuck out to me was that many women suffer from backache afterward. This is a perfect example of building the fancy house and skipping the laying of the foundations. Just because something now looks pretty from the outside doesn't mean that it is strong OR that you can skip that step and hope for the best. Many of these women will go away and do sit-ups with their nice new flat tummy and yes, it would look good, but the backache that they decide to live with because it is a by-product of 'looking' better is a warning sign they choose to ignore. What happens to these women down the track I am not sure, but I know it would be my recommendation that all of these women skip the sit-ups for a while (if not forever) and work within the guidelines of rebuilding from the inside out.

Down-training Obliques

I believe that when working well your TA (running horizontally) can help to bring your separation back together. I have worked with many women and found this to be a very effective way of fixing separation. BUT I will stress that it will only be effective if you are working your TA well and without the activation of your obliques. Through our experience we have learned that if you are continually activating TA with obliques they can actually counteract the joining process. TA may be working super hard to bring your abdominals back together but when challenged by obliques (which are often stronger anyway), responsible for twisting, they can actually counteract what you are doing and you may see little or no progress. This alone can hinder the rebuilding process, as it can be very disheartening when you are putting in a lot of effort and seeing no results.

A classic illustration of this was a mother who came to me with a four finger gap and was seemingly doing all of the right rebuilding exercises. BUT when we took a closer look and put her under Real Time Ultrasound we discovered that with every TA breath (the basic and first exercise we teach) she was not only activating her TA but also her obliques. Her TA was, every time, battling what is in most people a stronger and more dominant muscle. When we showed this to her and taught her how to activate her TA without obliques, we soon started to see progress and her separation improved dramatically in a relatively short period of time.

The main building block to fixing your abdominal separation is to really nail your TA breathing. By learning to do this well and without oblique activation you will learn to recruit your abdominals from the inside out. You will lay strong and sturdy foundations, and with these foundations you can go on to achieve way more within your exercise regime than you ever would if you just did sit-ups. By recruiting from the inside out I work with mothers who can hold a plank position for longer than four minutes. Please don't attempt this if you are yet to go through the rebuilding process, but I use it as an example of what you can achieve if you take the time now. I like to think that after having a baby we have this wonderful opportunity to really take the time and build our bodies properly. There are not many moments in your life where you feel it is acceptable to slow down, do gentle exercise and spend time on the simple stuff. After giving birth, your body is recovering in so many ways. I would love to empower you to embrace this time and do the really simple exercises that can also be quite relaxing, and do them really well. You will be setting yourself a fantastic foundation to not only achieving more amazing things through your health and fitness, but also taking great steps to avoid many of the common aches and pains that don't have to go hand in hand with motherhood.

> # Aches and pains don't have to come hand in hand with motherhood

How to Activate from the Inside Out

I will guide you through how to activate your abdominals from the inside out. However, like any exercise, learning from a book can be much less effective than in person. With this in mind, you can watch me on YouTube while I take you through this exercise. I also recommend that even once you have done this, and even if you think you have got it right, that you spend a little time and a little money on working with a health professional who has access to Real Time Ultrasound and can really let you know what you are doing. Real Time Ultrasound is a great visual tool as it means that you can see what you are doing on a screen. Sometimes women work well with audio cues, but I have seen amazing differences in awareness of activation when you can actually see what you are doing, so you know that when you do this it activates this muscle and when you do that it activates another. We can then fine tune the correct firing pattern and have you well on your way to rejoining your separation and discovering the tummy that you want to achieve.

Visit www.youtube/JenDugard for a video explanation of this exercise

- Start lying on your back
- Knees are bent and feet are hip width apart
- There is a straight line running from hips down to ankles so knees are not knocking in or falling out to the side
- Relax your shoulders
- Your spine is in neutral, so avoid over-arching of the lower back or pushing it into the ground
- Take one hand and place it on one of your obliques – you will find this just underneath your rib cage towards the side of your torso
- If you do a little cough or move from side to side you will feel your oblique pop up. Now you have felt it activate and know where it is – you can keep your hand on it but you don't want to feel it activate again

How to love your body as much as your baby

- Take your other hand and lay it from hipbone to hipbone or across your undies line (assuming you are wearing low-rise undies of course) – this is the area you are going to concentrate on throughout this exercise
- When you are ready, take a natural breath in, breathe all the way out and then draw in and up through your pelvic floor (I use the very glamorous analogy of imagining you have a tampon inserted and you are gently trying to squeeze it in and up when talking about a pelvic floor activation – remember to keep bum and back passage relaxed)
- Once you have got your pelvic floor contraction right we can move on to add your TA activation
- Take your natural breath in and as you breathe out gently draw your pelvic floor in and up then start to peel the skin away from your undies line towards your tailbone to activate your TA

This is a gentle movement and is generally about a lot less than what you may think you should be doing. There is no big 'tensing' or 'bracing' of the abdominals.

> # TA activation is a gentle contraction rather than a bracing movement

If you feel your obliques pop up or activate at any time, you should pull back and try your TA activation breath a little more gently. In time, as you become more familiar with the feeling and you are able to keep your obliques nice and relaxed, you will feel more connection to your TA. You will have the ability to bring it on more strongly and hold for a longer period of time and perform more challenging exercises, all by using your inner unit and while laying solid foundations, rather than relying on the fancy house. Remember it is important to acknowledge the feeling and the ability to completely relax your pelvic floor also.

At the beginning of this exercise perform some breaths where you activate pelvic floor and TA and completely relax between each breath. As we mentioned earlier, there is research to connect a hypertonic (overactive) pelvic floor to backache, so given learning all of this is partly designed to help you avoid backache, becoming aware of the relaxation phase of this exercise is essential.

When to Start

Most new mums are told that they need to wait until their six-week check-up to commence any exercise. This is true – I certainly don't recommend you get out and put yourself through any strenuous workouts prior to that, and even at the six-week mark you need to be gentle with yourself and remember that it is still very early days. I recommend longer after a caesarean section. However the breathing exercise I explained above is a

How to love your body as much as your baby

great way to start the process of rebuilding from the inside out, regaining awareness of your pelvic floor and TA. You can begin whenever you feel ready. If you can designate a little pelvic floor and TA time in between rocking and feeding and cuddling it would be fantastic. You will start the routine of ensuring you are doing something for yourself. I remember the days where you don't even manage time to have a shower. When you are experiencing this, if you are able to catch yourself, talk to your partner or support network and tell them you need even just 15 minutes a day to begin with to start working with yourself.

Remember quality over quantity

Remember that quality over quantity is vital when it comes to your pelvic floor exercises. Knowing you are doing your pelvic floor and transversus abdominis exercises correctly is the most important thing. Taking yourself to a quiet place where you can really tune in will always help this – it will also allow you a little headspace and time out.

If you haven't done it already upon the advice in this book, once you have had your six-week check-up with your midwife or obstetrician then, if possible, make the appointment with your chosen women's health physio. Find out exactly what is going on, on the inside, and work with that to begin your journey to becoming the strongest and fittest you have ever been AND achieving YOUR best ever body.

Essential Postural Exercises

From my work with lots of pregnant and postnatal mums, I know that along with abdominals, there are two other vital postural muscles that get lazy, and we need to take the time to activate and build strength there ahead of anywhere else. Once you have mastered your TA activations you can also target your glutes and your back and add a few simple exercises to your daily routine.

During pregnancy we carry most of our additional weight in our abdomen and breasts; our baby grows and our tummy gets heavier and boobs get bigger! Most women end up with a slight forward posture and a closing of the angle at the hips, tight hip flexors and more relaxed glutes, and a more forward posture in the upper body with rounded shoulders and tighter chest muscles. Sometimes, as a result of tight hip flexors and this forward posture, the glutes don't actually work properly anymore. Add to these tight or overactive hamstrings and the muscles in your bum become so inactive that they waste away, leaving you with a flatter backside than prior to pregnancy.

Many women complain of tightness around the neck area and aches across the upper back, and sometimes they are unable to properly stand upright any more. Once your baby is born, you spend even more time in this forward posture, rocking, carrying and breastfeeding, so this hunched look is ingrained even further and we have to work to open up the chest once again.

How to love your body as much as your baby

For tight hip flexors and a lazy bum:

Stretch: Hip Flexors

Strengthen: Glutes

In order to help to get those glutes firing again there are some simple exercises that you can do to help them along.

I recommend you visit my YouTube channel **www.youtube/ JenDugard** for a video explanation of these exercises

Stretch Hip Flexors

First up we need to stretch out your tight hip flexors – this can be done in either a standing or kneeling position.

Standing Hip Flexor Stretch

- Stand on one leg with a slight bend in the standing leg
- Bend the other leg behind you and hold it with one hand

- Pull your foot as close your to hamstring as possible
- Tuck your pelvis underneath and squeeze your glutes to feel your hip flexor stretching
- Hold for 20-30 seconds

Kneeling Hip Flexor Stretch

- Kneel down on your right knee – make sure it is on something soft
- Find a chair, couch or Swiss ball to put your right foot up on to– make sure this knee stays directly underneath the hip
- Tuck the pelvis underneath and squeeze your glutes to intensify the hip flexor stretch
- Reach up and over with the right arm
- Swap sides to use the left arm and leg
- Hold for 20-30 seconds

Strengthen Glutes

Hip Raise

- Lie flat on your back
- Knees bent, feet flat on the floor and hands by your side
- Have a little awareness through your TA
- Push down through your heels
- Squeeze your bum and raise your hips up to the sky

How to love your body as much as your baby

- You are aiming for a straight line from shoulders to ankles
- Squeeze and hold for 3-2-1
- Slowly lower down
- Repeat 10-12 times

If you feel your back at the top of this exercise don't go up quite so high – concentrate on feeling it through glutes rather than lower back.

> # Stretch the tight and strengthen the weak

Stretch: Chest

Strengthen: Back

No one wants to walk around in a hunched position with aching shoulders and upper back – by stretching out your chest muscles and strengthening your rhomboids (the ones that sit between your shoulder blades) you can start to combat and correct this posture.

In order to help to help you stand tall again there are some simple exercises that you can do:

Stretch Chest

- Place one against the edge of a wall or door frame
- Start down low and turn away from your hand to feel the stretch
- Hold for 3-2-1
- Turn in, move your hand to shoulder height, turn away
- Hold for 3-2-1
- Turn in, move your hand above your head, turn away
- Hold for 3-2-1

Strengthen Back

Cobra – can be done lying or standing

Lying Cobra

- Lie face down on the ground on a towel, hands down by your sides and chin and nose into towel, palms face down, legs and glutes relaxed with toes turned in
- As you breath out draw shoulders back and down
- Raise your upper body slowly off the floor
- Raise hands and turn thumbs up to the sky
- Squeeze shoulder blades together and keep trapezius relaxed
- Hold for a count of 3-2-1 and relax down to the ground
- Repeat 10-12 times

How to love your body as much as your baby

Standing Cobra

- Stand with feet hip width apart, chest up and shoulders down
- Have an awareness of your activation through your pelvic floor and TA
- Keeping the back straight, tip at the hips till fingertips are on knees
- As you breath out, lead with the thumbs, draw shoulders back and down and take arms behind you
- Turn thumbs up and squeeze shoulder blades together
- Hold for a count of 3-2-1 and relax back to start position
- Make sure back is still straight and chest is up
- Repeat 10-12 times

The great thing about these gentle yet effective exercises is that you can start them as soon as you feel ready. By combining your pelvic floor and TA activation exercises, your glute and back strengthening, hip flexor and chest stretching you will be reactivating all of the foundation muscles you need to ensure you build that good strong base, and be ready for the more challenging strengthening and exercise that is to come in your quest to discover your best ever body.

Body Before Baby

In an ideal world I would get this book into the hands of as many of you as humanly possible *before* you have your baby, either in pregnancy or even better, preconception. Imagine being armed with all of these tools and all of this knowledge before your world is turned upside down and your number one priority is no longer you. If you do happen to be one of those lucky women who is reading this book before your bub has come along, then taking action now can really make a difference to your post birth recovery and rebuild. I will talk later about preparation and consistency being key to achieving your goals and the word preparation couldn't fit here any better. If you have the opportunity to really prepare your body for childbirth, it is extremely valuable. I have seen cases of women who are pregnant presenting with abdominal separation, and through working with them during pregnancy we have been able to either stop the separation getting any worse, or even improve it with the correct exercises.

> ## Give this book to a
> ## pregnant mum you know

How to love your body as much as your baby

My Preconception or Pregnancy Check List

Be Active and Build Strength – if you have been exercising your whole life then this is fantastic; keep it up and ensure that you have a strength or resistance component to your routine – you may very well be grateful for all of those squats when you find yourself in that position during labour.

Know your Pelvic Floor and Transversus Abdominis – there is nothing saying that you must have already had a baby before you undergo Real Time Ultrasound to assess your pelvic floor contraction (and the ability to release – it's very useful if you can understand this bit before trying to push a baby out). Knowing how to activate your TA and down-train your obliques during or prior to pregnancy may also help to prevent additional abdominal separation.

Know what exercise is beneficial and which you should avoid – you can start this process by giving up sit-ups. Anything that may strengthen the rectus abdominus and creates pressure to your abdominal wall through flexion should be laid to rest for a while. In fact, say your goodbyes to sit-ups in general, as they may never become part of your exercise routine again (especially if I have anything to do with it). If you are pregnant, now isn't the time to begin any exercise that your body is not used to. Contact sports and sports such as horse riding are best avoided, along with ones that require a lot of balance and stability. Your centre of gravity will change as your baby grows and there may be more risk of falling.

Work with someone who knows their stuff – if you are a gym bunny and you don't feel comfortable doing your own research into what is and isn't recommended to include in your training program, now is a really great time to seek out a personal trainer or training group specialising and experienced in working with pre- and postnatal women. Ensuring you are doing the correct things now can really make a difference later on. It can offer great peace of mind knowing that you have an extra support person or group who can take you through pregnancy and beyond. I urge you to check the credentials of the person you choose to work with. After all, if you have a problem with your teeth you would not go to see and ear, nose and throat specialist, would you? You would seek out the best dentist you could find to fix up your teeth. It is up to you to do your research and work with the best possible person for you.

I said earlier not to commence any exercise that your body is not used to during pregnancy. I do see a lot of women who have fallen pregnant, not done much exercise in the past but have now decided that they need to get fit – during pregnancy. If you fall into this category and have taken yourself into a gym environment for the first time in years, it is great that you want to stay fit and healthy during your pregnancy but I would highly recommend that you seek out a health professional who can guide you through this time. It is more about what you can do rather than what you can't do, but again, knowing that you are in safe hands gives you great peace of mind.

Top Tips for Exercise during Pregnancy

Maintain rather than gain – Remember you are now in a maintenance phase rather than one of achieving any new goals or personal bests within your exercise program.

Rate yourself – Working to a Perceived Rate of Exertion (PRE) of seven out of 10 is recommended, with one being 'sitting on the couch and doing nothing' and 10 being 'can't possibly do any more'.

Stay cool – Monitor your temperature during exercise; your internal temperature is higher than your external and your baby has no way of cooling themself down. Prolonged periods of raised temperatures may cause harm – it may be worth skipping those hot yoga sessions or spin classes for a while.

Low impact – Concentrate on low impact exercise at this time; some women continue to run during pregnancy and everyone is different, but now is not the time to take up running. Remember, every time you run your pelvic floor is under more stress, so if you feel any kind of weakness or incontinence it may be time to stop for a while.

Stay stable – Be aware of changes in your centre of gravity; as that exercise you may have found easy last week becomes more difficult, you should also avoid lying flat on your back after the first trimester so as not to put pressure on the vena cava and decrease blood flow.

To lunge or not to lunge – This provides a point of debate amongst many fitness professionals. My advice would be that if your exercise program has contained lunges prior to you becoming pregnant, and you are fit and strong and you are not experiencing any pelvis or sciatic pain, you may be fine to continue to do lunges with a low weight through your pregnancy. Remember, however, if you start to feel any pelvic related pain or discomfort you should choose another leg exercise at this time. And certainly if you have never done a lunge before in your life, now is not the time to start.

Exercise is good – In most cases staying active and exercising through your pregnancy is of benefit to both mother and baby. HOWEVER, if you feel strange or unwell at any point, now is not the time to push on through. Stop what you are doing and seek the advice of your health or medical professional.

Introducing Jo Murdoch

I have worked with Jo since founding Body Beyond Baby. Jo and her team at The Physiotherapy Clinic have become an essential part of the care I offer to the women who I work with.

Jo is mum to her beautiful one-year old daughter, has 10 years experience and has a strong interest in treating women through pregnancy and the postnatal period. She is passionate about helping women rehabilitate their bodies post pregnancy and birth to return to their chosen exercise and sport. Jo holds a Bachelor of Physiotherapy (Honours), Post Graduate Certificate in Continence and Women's Health and is a director of The Physiotherapy Clinic.

Jo's top 5 expert tips when it comes to Rebuilding from the Inside Out

Treat the postnatal period as a rehabilitation period – it is crucial to your long-term wellbeing to strengthen what is weak. Take the time to have a postnatal assessment and rebuild areas of your body like your pelvic floor or abdominal wall properly from the beginning.

Return to exercise slowly – don't expect to bounce back to your training regime from before pregnancy and birth, respect that your body has had some time off exercise and needs to rebuild slowly.

Know your limits and stick to them – if you have been given advice on what your limits with exercise are, or are following the instructions in this book, ensure you do follow this advice as you will be grateful in the future when you are injury free, strong and fit.

Don't ignore the signs of pelvic floor dysfunction – please don't put up with urine or faecal leaking, heaviness through your pelvis, pelvic pain, painful intercourse, frequency with urine or bowel motion, constipation and or straining to open your bowels. There are people that are here to help you.

Exercise Exercise Exercise – if you're reading this book its likely you love to exercise. As physio's it's our business to keep people moving; we all know the benefits and done safely postnatally, it's brilliant for your body, mind, and baby!

More from Jo

Pregnancy and birth have the potential to change your posture, your pelvic floor function, your core stability and your motor control. Approximately 45 percent of women experience pelvic girdle pain in pregnancy, 62 percent of pregnant women have lumbo pelvic pain in the second trimester and 66 percent of women have a diastasis of the rectus abdominus by the third trimester.

Considering the impact pregnancy and birth can have on a women's body, it is essential the postnatal period is viewed as a time for structured, individualised rehabilitation. Our body is extremely clever at compensating for inadequacies in our neuromuscular system. Unfortunately, you can get about with these compensations free of symptoms for some time, before the compensations themselves start to fail. For example, Wilson et al., (2003), found 31 percent of women who did not have urinary incontinence in the early postnatal period reported urinary incontinence when assessed seven years post-partum.

There is strong evidence that has been pieced together in the last decade to demonstrate the link between incorrect motor patterns, lumbar spine pain, pelvic girdle pain, breathing dysfunction and stress urinary incontinence.

Ideally rehabilitation begins as soon as possible, to re-educate your body after pregnancy and birth and before your body has had time to consolidate incorrect motor patterns. It is highly recommended that you visit your physiotherapist, ideally one with a thorough understanding of women's health and core stability. Many physiotherapists who treat women during the postnatal period have access to a Real Time Ultrasound. With a Real Time Ultrasound you can see the muscles of the core and pelvic floor, how they contract independently of other muscles and how they contract during functional tasks. It also a fantastic tool to help teach you to use muscles appropriately again if dysfunction is identified.

Real Mums

Robin, mum to Jason(29), Jade(11) and Joshua(5)

I had my eldest son at 21. I had youth on my side and just seemed to bounce back. I then had my daughter when I was 39, and she is turning 12 this year. It was a natural birth and the labour took about two hours, so nothing too traumatic. During the pregnancy I did some prenatal yoga and swimming but always struggled with constant urinary tract infections. I understood a little bit about the pelvic floor muscles and the separation of the abdominals but didn't understand you had to retrain to get it back into shape.

After the birth of my daughter my main exercise was walking, lots of walking, 40 minutes to one hour of up and down hills. I went back into full-time work behind a desk and not much time for exercise. Any attempts I did try at exercise I found I wet myself, so I would just give it up. I just accepted this was my fate and didn't think too much of it. I would have days where I had hay fever and would be sneezing and wet myself. If I was at home I would be changing my underwear two to three times a day. If I was out I would just stop and cross my legs and brace myself for the sneeze and hope for the best. At 45 I had a lovely surprise and found out I was pregnant again, with my son. With this pregnancy I didn't do yoga but did do lots of swimming and walking. I also experienced more pelvic pains in the later stage of pregnancy, just due to the pressure, and so this limited the big long walks. At 39 weeks the doctors decided I should be induced due to my age and after 24 hours plus and what felt like hours of pushing, my son was born.

He was born posterior, or the wrong way round, which is why I had so much trouble pushing him out. In the end the doctor had to push him back in, reposition his head and help pull him out. It all happened very quickly. My poor baby had a big bruise on his head from hitting against my pelvis. From there everything seemed like a normal recovery and don't remember too much about my check-ups, just that I was told everything was okay. When my son was one-year old I decided to lose some weight, get fit and healthy. I joined a gym and saw a personal trainer twice a week. I was doing sit-ups among other exercises without any consideration to my pelvic floor or abdominal muscles. I found out later these weren't helping my separation or my weak pelvic floor. I also went to a naturopath and told her about my embarrassing flatulence. I was put on a diet and took some herbs to help with digestion. There wasn't much improvement but I stayed positive, hoping it would all come good.

After six months of trying the diet and 12 months with the personal trainer I gave it all away. I decided I would just go back to my old passion of running and took my daughter with me to compete in a cross-country club. It started at 2pm in the afternoon and I didn't think twice about it. Anyway, it was good fun at the start and I encouraged my daughter to run with me as she hadn't run two kilometres before.

But about 400metres into the run, urine just started to trickle out and I had no control over it at all. Since I was encouraging her to run I didn't want to stop. At the end of the race I tied a jumper around my waist and was so embarrassed, I couldn't wait to get out of there. I found when I would jog in the morning straight after getting out of bed I was fine but since this run was in the afternoon, after drinking water throughout the day, it was a different story. I never went back to the cross-country club.

I did all the common things too, like brace myself when I sneezed to make sure I didn't have any leakage. Last September I decided to look for an outdoor fitness class. I wanted to lose 10 kilos and had just turned 50. I wanted to be fit again. A friend of mine recommended Body Beyond Baby's 8 Week Challenge. I thought that would be fun to train with a friend and I went along, found the sessions fun and the support of all the other ladies kept me motivated. I remember the runs around the oval, which were 800metres. I tried my hardest not to have any 'accidents'. I would make sure I went to the toilet before, just in case, but still I would have some leakage towards the end of the run and would just run straight to the toilet again after. I kept persevering and just thought it has to come good, maybe I would take my last drink two hours before and limit my water intake during the session. I tried all sorts of tricks and even thought of wearing a sanitary pad, but just couldn't bring myself to do that. Luckily we were all ladies there so I wasn't too embarrassed. I went to sessions four times a week and at the start we always did the pelvic floor breathing exercise. I never thought too much of this until I also went to along to one of their pelvic floor and core workshops and saw via an ultrasound exactly what my pelvic floor was doing. It was through my training with Body Beyond Baby that I also found out it wasn't okay to leak during running, exercise or in life in general. I really thought it was just my fate after having three children. I became more enthusiastic and started doing my pelvic floor exercises before I went to bed. One day when I was running I was bracing myself for some leakage but it didn't happen. Then I became a bit cheeky and even drank a glass of water before a run and who knew... still no leakage. I have also noticed the embarrassing flatulence has all but gone. It has taken six months to retrain my pelvic floor and now when I train I don't have to worry – I am so happy about this. It feels like I have a new skill.

My daughter is turning 12 this year and all that time I had just accepted my fate that leakage was just the norm. Then my son came along, just adding to the weakness. Now, after six months of training, I can confidently have a drink of water before I run. How good is that! I will do another follow up with Jo (physiotherapist) to be completely confident I know what's going on, on the inside. I have also lost five kilos on my journey and increased my core strength and stability, which I believe has also taken some pressure off my pelvic floor.

Rebekah, mum to Noah(2.5) and Ivy(3m)

Falling pregnant in January 2010 with our son Noah was an amazing and life changing experience for my husband and I. Having always led a healthy lifestyle before falling pregnant, it was important for me to maintain my fitness while pregnant and beyond.

Throughout my first pregnancy, I continued with my boot camp training up until 10 weeks into my pregnancy. At this time I decided to stop this style of exercise, as this specific camp was not designed for expectant mums. For the remainder of the pregnancy I continued to walk everyday and continued with body strength exercises throughout.

Our son Noah was born on 13 October 2010. The labour was quick, however the pushing phase lasted more than two hours. Due to the force of this and being left with a second degree tear, I was suffering from bladder leakage. Post birth, I found I would leak when the shower was turned on or when flushing the toilet (thinking I was finished) would also create a leakage issue.

I was introduced to Body Beyond Baby through my mothers group. It was now three months since the birth of Noah and I was beginning to see beyond the fatigue and wanted to start taking care of my body and mind once again. I began attending sessions regularly two days a week. When completing the required paperwork one of the questions asked was about pelvic floor and leakage. I thought twice about how to answer this one; do I be honest and admit to it? It's embarrassing and

How to love your body as much as your baby

surely it will fix over time. However, I admitted I was suffering from leakage. Upon attending my first class, Jen took the time to discuss these issues with me. She advised that I would need to visit a women's health physio in relation to my pelvic floor weakness and provided details of Jo Murdoch from the Physiotherapy Clinic. Until I was able to visit Jo and we understood the situation, I was unable to run in the sessions. My initial reaction to this was what? 'What do you mean I can't run? I am fit, I trained through my pregnancy – what am I paying for if I am unable to get a complete workout? 'I left that first session rather frustrated by Jen's suggestion and did not understand the real issues.

Within a couple of weeks I was able to meet with Jo, who confirmed that I was suffering from a very weak pelvic floor, which had been damaged through the birthing process. After assessing me through Real Time Ultrasound, she was able to reassure me that by taking the time to complete the appropriate pelvic floor exercises and gently taking the time in the exercise classes to rebuild, I could be back running within a month or so. Three sessions with Jo and I was given the green light to introduce running again.

Jen's philosophy of taking the time to rebuild from the inside out I could not agree with more. Having to deal with the initial frustrations of a slow road to recovery I became fitter and stronger than I had ever been before.

After 14 months of training with Body Beyond Baby I found out I was pregnant with my second child. Again, it was important that I was able to keep training throughout the pregnancy and having found Body Beyond Baby, this was possible. Having regained all of my pelvic floor stability by rebuilding my inner unit meant that I was able to train up until 37 weeks with my second child.

On 16 January 2013 our daughter Ivy was born. Because my inner core unit was a lot stronger I had a quick recovery after the birth. After my six-week postnatal check was completed, I was back in the park training again. I believe this was due to the guidance and professional advice offered by Jen and her team.

A revisit to Jo at the Physiotherapy Clinic following the birth of Ivy, confirmed my pelvic floor required some work to get it back to 100 percent but it was definitely stronger than after my first pregnancy.

To quote Jen, if you find out exactly what is going on in the inside and work with that to begin your journey, you can become the strongest and fittest you have ever been and achieve your best ever body. I believe this is what happened for me and I look forward to the same journey following my second child. Thanks Jen!

5 Easy to Implement Actions

1. Know how to activate and relax your pelvic floor and know how to do it well!

2. Check for abdominal separation

3. Learn how to activate your TA

4. Learn and implement our simple posture exercises

5. See a Women's Health Physio for a full assessment using Real Time Ultrasound if possible

Exercise – Part 2

Building the Fancy House

This could be seen as the fun bit, the exciting bit – it's often the bit that most fitness books are *just* about. You know, what exercise should be done on what day, pictures, diagrams, reps and sets. You will find some of that here but, as I hope you have already discovered, this book is not about quick fixes or just showing you how to build the fancy house. It is about long-term change and the best and most effective ways to build the strongest, fittest and sexiest body you have ever had – all while having children in tow.

If you are one of those super enthusiastic people who has decided to get stuck into your new exercise regime and you have picked up this book and skipped straight to the bit that talks about what you look like on the outside, I'm sure that 'Building the Fancy House' is way more appealing to some of you than 'Rebuild from the Inside Out'. If that is you, be honest with yourself. I am now going to ask you to flip back to part one of this chapter entitled 'Rebuild from the Inside Out'. If this is you and you feel a little disappointed that you're not going to get down to the nitty gritty just yet, let me tell you that THAT is the nitty gritty – THAT chapter is your key to achieving your best body yet. Skip that stage and you could find yourself in the long line of mothers who are suffering from all of the aches and pains that don't have to go hand in hand with motherhood. Make the decision now to go on a different journey, not one of quick fixes; overexercising and crash diets because you just want things to happen quickly. We've all been there in our past but now is the time to allow your body the time it needs to rebuild itself (with your help, of course). Let go of the woman who wanted everything now – you've just spent nine months growing a baby. The ultimate in delayed gratification, in a world where we want everything right now, there's no rushing the nine months it takes for you to meet your baby, even longer from the time you decided you wanted a baby, so resist the urge to rush your post baby body. It also took your body nine months to change into what it is now, so it only makes sense that we give it time and love to change into something new.

I'd also like to stress here that it's not always about the way we look. For many women it's what their body can do that is important to them. Being able to run around with your children may very well be more important to you than the way you look in the mirror. Knowing that you can be fitter and healthier than ever before, that you can still run and feel exhilarated, can

How to love your body as much as your baby

achieve something new within your fitness routine. We then find a by-product of being active is that the body naturally will follow.

We are all on our own journey

For some it will take longer than others. It can even vary from pregnancy to pregnancy for the same mother. I found the post baby body journey different after both of my pregnancies. I had each journey documented; along with body composition scans at regular intervals after each of my children was born. What I found quite interesting was that on both occasions, exactly one year after the births I was at the same body fat percentage (notice here I talk about body fat and not weight – more on that later). However, at the three-month mark after my first pregnancy I had made much more progress in losing the weight than in my second. Second time around the journey seemed to take longer, and if I hadn't had my baseline measurements and so known where I was starting from and the progress I was making, it may have been quite frustrating. This is a great instance both of how important it is to start your journey with some solid figures, and also of how your journey can vary from pregnancy to pregnancy, let alone woman to woman.

So assuming you are now onto the right chapter, that you have at least read Rebuild from the Inside Out and you have a plan of action, then lets get started.

Knowing Where you are Coming From

You might not want to accept or put solid measurements on what the last nine months has done to you (or how those endless packets of Tim Tams didn't just disappear when your baby came out). I encourage you to make the decision to allow yourself to accept where you are right now. As well as knowing where you would like to be and what YOUR best ever body looks like, you need to know exactly where you are starting from. There are going to be times when this journey is hard and times where you feel like you are making progress on a daily basis. The importance of tracking your progress is vital at both of these times. We need to know what's working and what's not, pick you up when you feel like it's all happening too slowly (because in my experience, even at those times things aren't usually as bad or as slow as they seem). We need to be able to celebrate your progress and know when you have reached your goal (don't worry, you can always move the goal posts and adapt your journey).

Forget about Weight

When we talk about losing weight it can be very misleading. Yes, the majority of you will want to see the number on the scales get smaller, but there will be times when if you rely solely on the number on the scales you will never know the true picture of what is happening on the inside. I am sure many of you have heard that muscle weighs more than fat, but our female brains can find it hard to get over the fact that once you start to exercise and become fitter and stronger, that number might never get back down to where it was before. That's not to say you cannot be as lean or possibly even leaner than you have been in the past, just that your body composition may have changed. Let's take a quick look at my own example that I spoke about at the beginning of this book and how my body composition has changed over the years.

Date of Scan	Time in life	Body fat %	Total Body Weight (kg)	Fat Mass (kg)	Lean Body Mass (kg)
May-07	Just after wedding	16.9	49.9	8.4	39.3
Sep-08	2m after 1st baby	27.2	58.6	15.9	40.4
Dec-08	5m after 1st baby	22.5	55.3	12.4	40.6
Jul-09	12m after 1st baby	21.3	55.5	11.8	41.3
Sep-10	2m after 2nd baby	30.0	61.8	18.5	40.9
Dec-10	5m after 2nd baby	28.3	59.9	16.9	40.5
Jul-11	12m after 2nd baby	21.7	54.8	11.9	40.5
Nov-11	16m after 2nd baby	16.6	54.4	9.0	43.0

So here is your license to really get over the number on the scales. I won't lie, it definitely took me a while, especially this year when I have put on more weight in muscle, so I saw the number actually creep up instead of down, despite body fat staying at a similar level. But it's pretty liberating when you reach a point where that number doesn't define you any more.

Ways to Measure your Progress

Scales – measure just weight; probably the most widely used tool but certainly not the most effective. There are lots of variables with only using the scales, for example; water retention and hydration, last night's meal, etc.

Tape measure – a great tool to use in conjunction with the scales and you will discover you are getting smaller, but again, by measuring alone it is hard to know what is going on, on the inside. You can do this at home using the following sites for measurement; chest (be aware that when breastfeeding, the chest measurement isn't a reliable one), waist (the smallest part), middle (the bit that crosses your belly button), hips (at the widest part, usually about crotch level), thigh (make sure you choose the same spot to measure each time), arm relaxed, arm flexed (this one is great as you want to see the number of the relaxed arm going down but the number of the flexed arm going up, to see you are putting on muscle).

Skin folds – done with callipers, you would need to seek out a fitness professional who uses callipers within their testing routine. When used in conjunction with scales and measurements, so long as testing remains consistent, you will be able to see fat mass (rather than just weight) dropping. I would advise you to work with the same person assessing your body fat levels using callipers throughout your journey. Testing can vary from person to person and you could end up with very different

How to love your body as much as your baby

results, but if you stick to just one person you should hopefully see the numbers getting smaller and testing will remain more consistent. The biggest revelation here is when you see the numbers on the scale remain the same, yet the numbers for your skin folds are falling.

DEXA scan – this is my most highly recommended tool and one I use with all of my personal training clients. There is no arguing with what your DEXA scan says. There are no variables and it will tell you your exact body composition; fat mass, muscle mass, water, even bone density (which for females especially is great to know). Your DEXA scan will even tell you how much fat and muscle you have in your right arm in comparison to your left. I discovered through my own testing, both before and after my pregnancies, that my body put on muscle mass through my trunk during pregnancy and then this muscle dropped away when it was no longer needed to help carry the weight of my babies.

*Please visit my website **www.jendugard.com** to help you find where you can get a DEXA scan*

The Importance of Goal Setting

Before moving on to actual exercise we need to know what you would like to achieve. Just as when you plan your journey when getting into a car to go to a new destination, you need to plan your journey to discovering YOUR best ever body.

Yes, things may change along the way, you may need to stop for fuel at an unexpected destination, and I can guarantee the world of motherhood will throw you challenges and curve balls that threaten to throw you off track. But if you have a clear picture of what you are aiming for you, are much more likely to achieve your goals.

Alternative Measures and Motivations

By now you know where you are starting through using one of our suggested tools for baseline body measurements. You can also use other measures and motivations such as:

Get your old favourite jeans out and putting them somewhere you see them regularly – try them on and take a photo of what they look like on now (even if you can do them up at the moment). You might not like the idea now but I promise, when you have this image to look back on it will be a clear visual reminder on how far you have come – and one we often forget.

Take a before photograph – no one has to see it but you and you can take it yourself in the mirror then hide it away, but from my experience when your body starts to change you often forget just how far you have come without this visual reminder.

Find an image of the body you would like to achieve– put it somewhere you can see it often. This can either be a previous photograph of yourself or you could choose an image of someone you have found in a magazine or on the internet.

How to love your body as much as your baby

Perform actual fitness testing that covers strength, cardio and stamina – as much as you may be on a weight loss journey, this is also a journey to make you stronger and fitter than you have ever been (or as fit as YOU want to be).

Set your Targets

Then its time to start to get down to the nitty gritty: WHAT exactly YOU want to achieve and how you are going to do it. The clearer your goals, the easier it will be to picture your outcome and use this to drive your journey.

Tips for Goals setting:

Write your goal in the positive instead of the negative.

> **'I am wearing my favourite skinny jeans'**, rather than **'I don't want to wear my maternity clothes any more'**.

And in the present instead of future.

> **'I am wearing my favourite skinny jeans'**, rather than **'I will be wearing my favourite skinny jeans'**.

Make you Goals SMART.

> **S** = Specific
> **M** = Measurable
> **A** = Attainable
> **R** = Realistic
> **T** = Timely

Specific *is the What, Why and How* – What do you want to ultimately accomplish? Why is this important to do at this time? How are you going to do it? (By...)

Ensure the goals you set are very **specific, clear and easy.** Instead of setting a goal to lose weight or be healthier, set a specific goal to lose two centimetres off your waistline or to run five kilometres.

Measurable – *if you can't measure it, you can't manage it.* Choose a goal with measurable progress so you can see the change occur. How will you see when you reach your goal? Be specific! 'I will run five kilometres by June 1', shows the specific target to be measure. 'I want to be a good runner', is not as measurable.

Attainable – *a goal needs to stretch you slightly so you feel you can do it and it will need a real commitment from you.* The feeling of success that this brings helps you to remain motivated.

Realistic – *a realistic challenge should push you to make a real and lasting change, be a little uncomfortable at times,*

How to love your body as much as your baby

but it shouldn't break you. Set goals that you can attain with some effort! Too high and you set the stage for failure, but too low sends the message that you aren't very capable. **Set the bar high enough for a satisfying achievement!**

Time – *set a timeframe for the goal.* For next week, in three months – putting an end point on your goal gives you a **clear target** to work towards. This is where joining a group or teaming up with a friend to set yourselves an 8 Week Challenge or something similar can be very powerful. **Time must also be measurable, attainable and realistic.**

Now that you have figured out your destination, we need to make sure you a have a road map to get there. What is the best type of exercise for you? Are there types of exercise you should be avoiding? How often should you be exercising? What will be the most effective?

What Type of Exercise should You Choose?

Although there is no one size fits all scenario, I do know what has worked for me and what has worked for many of the mothers I have worked with. As we progress I will introduce you to what I have found to be the key information you can use as you move forward on your journey.

When embarking on an exercise program as a mother, it is especially important that you are aware of what you are doing and why. That you take the time to gain advice to ensure you are doing the safest and most effective workout for the time you have available. Gone are the days of leisurely hanging out in the gym and wandering around trying new pieces of equipment, having a chat and getting round to doing some exercise. You are now sleep deprived, short on time and looking for your best possible solution to achieve YOUR best ever body. You need to know what type of exercise to do, and a little bit about why you are doing it and what it is doing for you. With informed choices you can then work with a specialised personal trainer to tailor this to you even further, or you can at least start to understand how to put something together for yourself.

What are the choices?

To make it super simple, aside from your rebuilding or postural type exercise, we can break your exercise down into just two categories – cardiovascular and resistance.

Cardiovascular (cardio) exercise

Cardio is that which gets your heart rate up and should make you sweat.

When performing cardio exercise your body uses whichever source is easiest to burn. Given that muscle is easier for the body to use for energy than fat, you will often see people who only do cardio exercise are part of our fat skinny phenomenon, due to the fact that they are doing no exercise to maintain

How to love your body as much as your baby

or increase their muscle mass. Add to this the snowball effect of a decrease in muscle mass, slowing your metabolism, so when you start to eat more or stop doing so much cardio, you will put weight on more easily due to your body not needing to burn as much energy at rest as those with a higher percentage of muscle mass.

The other thing to remember about cardio – especially the long slow type which many people often go for first – is that you will only see changes for a relatively short amount of time. You go for your first run and it is hard – you might run for 15 minutes and feel exhausted. Next time you go out for 20 minutes, then 25, then 30 and because your body is working harder than it is used to, you will start to see changes. Your weight on the scales will be moving down, which is exactly what you think you want to see. Your body will be dropping fat BUT because you are only doing cardio it may also be losing muscle. To continue to see results you must either eat less (there's only a certain amount of food a person, especially a mum, can get down to and in my opinion its often WAY too little) or start to run more. Your 30 minute run becomes 35, then 40, 45 then 50 – before you know it you are running for an hour. Before we have even begun to talk about the daily wear and tear on your joints, you soon plateau and have to figure out how to find the time to run for longer so that you continue to see results. I am assuming you are like me – you certainly don't have much more than an hour in your day (if that) to spend long distance running. Add to the time issue the fact that when you are long distance running, although your body is burning energy during your exercise time, as soon as you stop it stops. How cool would it be to do exercise that has your metabolism firing long after the time that you actually finished?

Now I'm not saying don't do any cardio – I'm saying you need to do the right type of cardio and you need to complement it with resistance exercise.

Interval Training

To better your current routine of longer slower runs or other cardio, I suggest you change your cardio exercise (when you are ready) to interval training.

I am a big fan of interval training. With long slow cardio I get bored of just pounding the pavement, and when you have short-term goals to be working towards throughout it's much easier to get through your training session.

By performing intervals where you work harder for a shorter period of time then go into a recovery phase, your body will ultimately work harder and burn more energy than if you were to just do a long slow cardio workout.

For example you might start with:
- 1 min – work as hard as possible (Perceived Rate of Exertion or PRE 9-10)
- 2 min – recovery (PRE 5-6)
- Repeat for 20-30 mins depending on time allowed

How to love your body as much as your baby

Next workout you would then decrease the rest time:

- 1 min – work as hard as possible (PRE 9-10)
- 1 min 30 sec – recovery (PRE 5-6)
- Repeat for 20-30 mins depending on time allowed

Then decrease rest again:

- 1 min – work as hard as possible (PRE 9-10)
- 1 min – recovery (PRE 5-6)
- Repeat for 20-30 mins depending on time allowed

And again so the rest becomes shorter than the work time:

- 1 min – work as hard as possible (PRE 9-10)
- 45 sec– recovery (PRE 5-6)
- Repeat for 20-30 mins depending on time allowed

And again:

- 1 min – work as hard as possible (PRE 9-10)
- 30 sec– recovery (PRE 5-6)
- Repeat for 20-30 mins depending on time allowed

From here you can then increase work time and use the same theories, so you are continuing to challenge your body and make it work harder but you do not have to increase the actual time spent training. As a mum, you need to do the most efficient workout possible in the time you have available.

For example:

- 2 min – work as hard as possible (PRE 9-10)
- 2 min – recovery (PRE 5-6)
- Repeat for 20-30 mins depending on time allowed

Next session:

- 2 min – work as hard as possible (PRE 9-10)
- 1 min 30 sec – recovery (PRE 5-6)
- Repeat for 20-30 mins depending on time allowed

And so on.

As I mentioned before, we are all different and it can take a little while to figure out what works best for you. I have used the above training methods with many of the mums I work with who want to increase their fitness levels, drop body fat and have limited time available. Some of these women could not run at all when we started, but by starting off slow, increasing their work time and decreasing their rest time they are now much more comfortable running. I have given you a great starting point and something to work with, but feel free to tweak it and figure out what works best for you.

Remember to write down what you do each day. Not only will it help you to remember what you are up to so you can work harder next time, but it is really great to look back in a few weeks time at the progress you have made and how far you've come.

The other terrific thing about this type of workout is that you can translate it into any form of cardio you like. If you aren't ready to run yet you can swim, or if you enjoy rowing you can row.

Resistance Training

Resistance exercise is that which causes your body to react to the intensity of the exercise you are doing to make it stronger. Every time you do a resistance training session and you push your limits, some of your muscle fibres are broken down. Your body then knows that it needs to become stronger in order to be able to do the same thing more easily next time, so it rebuilds the broken muscle fibres, not to their original strength, but to stronger than before. This is why you can increase the number of reps you can do or weight you can lift over time.

Let's look at the benefits of resistance training:

The more muscle you carry the more energy your body needs to maintain itself at rest – this is called your metabolic rate. Increase your muscle mass and in turn your metabolism will increase and you will burn more fat.

As you age and especially as females we become more at risk of diseases such as osteoporosis – losing weight from walking and a calorie restricted diet alone can result in a decline of bone density. Resistance exercise over time actually increases your bone density, leaving you at much lower risk of developing osteoporosis in later life.

You will increase your strength and balance, enabling your muscles, tendons and joints to work more efficiently – therefore increasing their functionality, flexibility and stamina.

The decrease in muscle mass and unsteadiness that appears to be a natural result of getting older may not be quite so set in stone.

You will be warding off other diseases – such as cancer, heart disease, diabetes and also reducing the risk of injury.

You will become physically stronger – and able to carry out day-to-day activities, and that growing child, much more easily.

You will look firmer– and often have a more positive self-image.

You will feel healthier, have more energy and sleep more soundly – okay this one may depend upon some cooperation from your little one, but best get the right practices in place for the time that they sleep right through...wouldn't that be wonderful!

Avoid the Fat Skinny Phenomenon

We all have a different image of the body we would like to live in, but for your own inner strength and your body's ability to avoid injury and fetch and carry and run around after your children, here's one I recommend you avoid. If you discover you fall into this category, know that you now have the knowledge and the tools to do something about it.

Fat skinny may be a contradiction in terms but it definitely exists. Generally you see this in people that are just naturally skinny. They seemingly have no real reason to exercise because they're not fat. You look at their body from a side-on angle and the first thing that stands out (or doesn't) is a lack of a bum. It's basically a straight line from back to legs. They have no muscle tone or definition through their arms, and a word that might describe them is thin. This body type can generally eat whatever they like without gaining weight but although small, their body is soft and maybe even a little flabby. Many think it is lucky to have this kind of body type where you don't have to watch your weight, do little exercise, eat whatever you like and remain skinny. In my opinion these people are much more likely to be unhealthy for this very reason. They don't have the obvious warning signs, like fat gain, that the rest of us do to keep them in check, and they are definitely often more unhealthy on the inside than their more conscientious friends who are eating more healthily to watch their weight.

Let's look a little more about the secrets and myths of losing body fat rather than weight.

Stop JUST Walking

No, I didn't say stop walking, I said stop JUST walking; your body will use muscle for energy as well as burning fat if all you do is walk to lose weight. The typical fat skinny person's physique belongs to that of the serial walker who has never even looked at a dumbbell, let alone lifted one. Add some resistance training to your routine, build and maintain your muscle mass.

Weights will not make you look like a man

Quite the opposite. In fact, by adding the right resistance exercise to your fitness routine you will start to build muscle which will give you shape and tone in all of the right places. It is very hard for most women to put on the amount of muscle mass it would take for us to look big and bulky. The amount of food you would have to eat, and training you would have to commit to, prevents most women from ending up this way. What weight training will do, when done well, is to give you shape and tone in all of the right places. It will allow you to build upon that bum, which you now know how to activate from our Rebuild from the Inside Out chapter to stop it being saggy. It will give you toned thighs and definition through your arms, especially your triceps, which will help you to avoid the 'bingo wings' that seem to creep up on many women as they get older.

Resistance training will make you look firm and not floppy. Most women I know would definitely prefer firm over floppy!

By ensuring you have all muscles firing in the right order through your rebuild from the inside out process, and then by including weight training into your routine, you will be ensuring you stay out of the category of mums who have no bums and in that of sexy curves and backsides to be proud of!

Busy Mum Workout Must-knows!

Choose compound exercises

Just as I believe interval training is the best option for mum when it comes to cardiovascular training, I also have a favourite when it comes to resistance training. And my favourite type of resistance training comes in the form of compound exercises.

A compound exercise is one that uses more than one joint and more than one muscle group. For example, a squat would be an example of a compound exercise because it uses both the hip and knee joints, along with the glutes, hamstrings and quads to complete the movement. It then makes sense that there are exercises which you should stay clear of if you are aiming to do the most effective workout possible in a limited amount of time. These time wasting exercises are things like bicep curls or calf raises; isolated exercises that use just one joint and one muscle to perform.

Right up there with my absolute favourites are what I refer to as double compound exercises. These are like a super sized compound exercise that can often include two, three or even four joints and muscles groups. For example, a squat into an overhead press uses hips, and knees, hamstrings, quads and glutes for the squat element. Then to take the weight overhead you are using both your shoulder and your elbow joints and introducing deltoids and triceps within the same exercise – double whammy, and perfect for a busy mum.

I also know that in daily life we often don't have the luxury of controlled movements and are often using our whole bodies to lift, carry, change and lurch for one child while holding the door open for the other, so it is important that once we have solidified our foundations that we challenge the way we train and introduce varied movements in different directions, using lots of muscles and joints simultaneously.

Opposing muscle groups

Choose exercises to do one after the other that use the opposite muscle groups. This way you can work quickly, rest less and again complete the most time efficient workout while spending as much energy as possible.

Remember:

    If you PULL – you are working your back and biceps.

    If you PUSH – you are working your chest and triceps.

Put together as many variations as you like in order to work these muscle groups one after another and keep moving!

You can also switch between upper body and lower body exercises to gain the same effect.

Add cardio

Cardio will keep your heart rate up and keep you working harder, again using your time in the most effective way.

Legs are the exception

Your legs are much larger muscles and you can get away with loading them for more than one exercise in sequence. By choosing different exercises you will be targeting different parts of the legs.

Sample training programs

Your sample resistance training session may look like this:

*All of these training sessions can be found on **www.youtube. com/JenDugard***

***Program 1** – Using the upper body/lower body theory*

Squat x 12
Push-ups x 12
Cardio – 1 min

Sumo Squat x 12
Row x 12
Cardio – 1 min

Alternating Lunge x 12
Triceps Dips x 12
Cardio – 1 min

Step-ups x 12
Lat Pull-down x 12
Cardio – 1 min

Program 2 – Using opposing muscle groups (excluding legs)

Squat x 12
Static Lunge x 12 each leg
Cardio – 1 min

Push-ups x 12
Lat Pull-Down x 12
Cardio – 1 min

Triceps Dips x 12
Row x 12
Cardio – 1 min

Program 3 – Double Compound Exercises

Squat Row x 12
Squat Press x 12
Cardio – 1 min

Lunge with Single Arm Row x 12
Push-up into Side Prone x 12
Cardio – 1 min

Sumo Squat with Biceps Curl x12
Lunge with Single Arm Press x 12 each side
Cardio – 1 min

To help you get a feel for the routine you might want to put together for yourself, all of these training sessions can be found on my YouTube channel.

How to love your body as much as your baby

Your body was designed to move daily so it is my recommendation that you do exactly that. Remember to rest and allow your body recovery time but for the health and wellbeing of both you and your baby some activity on a daily basis is very important.

Your ideal ultimate weekly training program

- Monday – Compound resistance exercises.
- Tuesday – Cardio interval training.
- Wednesday – Compound resistance exercises.
- Thursday – Cardio interval training.
- Friday – Compound resistance exercises.
- Saturday – Other exercise that you enjoy, with no fixed structure, to keep your routine fun and interesting.
- Sunday – active recovery, take a leisurely stroll with your partner and/or baby.

This is a sample training program; it's up to you to work out what works best within your week and to build up to your own ideal program.

While you are doing your rebuilding exercises, and as you are starting to feel a little more normal again, you might start with one interval training session and one compound training session per week and just walk on the other days. Increase your scheduled exercise as you feel ready – there is no pressure, everyone is different, and there is no right or wrong.

Training to the Weakest Link

When starting your resistance routine it is important to know what is going on, on the inside so that you can work with any weaknesses to build your overall strength.

Find out, for example, if you have a weakened pelvic floor or abdominal wall. It is important to seek expert advice before you rush into high intensity exercise (many of us can get very overenthusiastic when we get started on a health kick); you could be doing yourself damage. I see many women who over-compensate, using one group of muscles to make up for the fact that the ones that should be working aren't doing their job properly. You are more likely to end up with injuries down the track and then get frustrated because all your hard work has gone to waste.

Knowing your weakest link is extremely valuable – only then can you ensure you are doing the safest and most effective exercise program for you.

Changes and checks

Here are a couple of common contraindications I see in many mums, along with simple checks you can do and adaptations you can implement to make sure you are training to your weakest link.

How to love your body as much as your baby

Weak pelvic floor

Having a weaker pelvic floor, at least initially, is very common after having a baby. If you know about it, look after it, do your personalised retraining program and adapt your general training – you will soon be back to normal. If you ignore it, you could end up suffering from incontinence by the time you turn 55. It's amazing how many older women I talk to who do struggle with incontinence issues, mostly because previously this subject hasn't been widely discussed – it's one of those traditional put up and shut-up subjects that used to be viewed as just an inevitable by-product of becoming a mum.

It is commonly thought that it is the only exercises that create impact that can cause a pelvic floor weakness to worsen. Although this is definitely the case with high impact exercises there are also other, lower impact and less recognised exercises that can also cause damage.

So how do you know if a certain type of exercise or movement is too hard or intense for your pelvic floor?

Exercise: Running

How to recognise a weakness:

Leakage of bladder or bowel, any feeling of heaviness, or it being different than before.

What to do:

- You need to listen to your body and stop running
- If you haven't had a pelvic floor check-up then make that first on your To-Do list. When you have this information you can then act with the advice of your health professional
- If you can activate your pelvic floor, but lack endurance, then stop/start running may still be okay for you; longer runs are best avoided
- If you cannot activate your pelvic floor at all, it may be that running is not the best exercise choice for you at this time

Exercise: Squat

How to recognise a weakness:

Leakage of bladder or bowel, any feeling of heaviness or it being different than before, losing sensation or the ability to contract and release during your squat.

Quick check:

- Start by ensuring you have the correct set-up with your feet a little wider than your hips and your weight through your heels

- When you get to the bottom of your squat hold it for a few seconds and see if you can contract and release your pelvic floor
- If you cannot contract and release at this point then this type of exercise, done to this intensity, is too hard for you right now

What to do:

- Decrease or get rid of any additional weight (dumbbells/resistance bands etc.)
- Repeat the quick check above
- IF you CAN now contract and release you can continue at this intensity
- IF you CAN'T – continue to make your squat easier by losing the weights all together or decreasing the range of motion (or depth) of your squat
- Stop at your reduced depth and try the contract and release test again
- Continue to do this until you have found a depth at which you can contract and release and know your pelvic floor is working

Exercise: Push-ups

How to recognise a weakness:

Leakage of bladder or bowel, any feeling of heaviness or it being different than before, losing sensation or the ability to contract and release during your push-up.

Quick check:

- Start by doing a push-up on your knees, making sure you have the correct set-up and alignment, with your hands directly beneath your shoulders
- As you lower down into your push-up, hold the position at the bottom (just before your chest reaches the ground) and see if you can contract and release your pelvic floor
- If you cannot contract and release your pelvic floor at this point then this type of exercise, done to this intensity, is too hard for you right now

What to do:

- Decrease intensity by dropping to your knees or, if you started on your knees, by placing your hands on a raised surface (i.e. a bench or step)
- Repeat the quick check above

How to love your body as much as your baby

- IF you CAN now contract and release you can continue at this intensity
- IF you CAN'T – continue to make your push-up easier by raising your hands further, or reduce the depth of your push-up
- Stop at your reduced depth and try the contract and release test again
- Continue to raise your hands to the point at which you can contract and release and know your pelvic floor is working
- If you cannot activate your pelvic floor at all in your push-up you might need to try an alternate exercise at this time (i.e. Chest Press where there is less intra-abdominal pressure due to not having to hold your body in a prone position)

Exercise: Prone hold

Many people think that a prone position is the perfect exercise to build strength through your core. However, a prone creates a considerable amount of intra-abdominal pressure that will push out through a weakened pelvic floor and abdominal wall; it should not be used as your go-to exercise for building core strength. Make sure you complete your rebuilding exercises prior to getting to this one.

How to recognise a weakness:

Leakage of bladder or bowel, any feeling of heaviness or it being different than before, losing sensation or the ability to contract and release during your prone

Quick check:

- Start by doing your prone hold on your knees, make sure you have the correct set-up and alignment, with your shoulders directly above your elbows
- As you hold your prone position see if you can contract and release your pelvic floor
- If you cannot contract and release your pelvic floor at this point then this type of exercise, done to this intensity, is too hard for you right now

What to do:

- Decrease intensity by moving straight away into an all fours position with your hands directly beneath your shoulders and your knees directly beneath your hips. Most women should be able to contract and release in this position
- Continue your rebuilding exercises to strengthen your pelvic floor before attempting your prone position again

How to love your body as much as your baby

I have chosen these examples as they are common exercises and often not considered damaging to your pelvic floor. But the rule of thumb is that anything which causes intra-abdominal pressure (makes you strain, requires effort or causes you to hold your breath) can be damaging to your pelvic floor, especially if it is already weak.

You can use the tests above during pretty much any exercise to check in and make sure all is working well and that the exercise you are doing is at a suitable level or intensity for you at this time; you may find that different exercises are better or worse for you. I have found that women who have pelvic floor control during a normal squat might struggle more during a sumo squat (due to being more stretched in a wider stance), and some women who find it hard to squat may be able to perform a static lunge instead.

Abdominal Separation or *Diastasis Recti*

Along with ensuring you are doing your rebuilding exercises, knowing that you have abdominal separation is a key part of your journey to building the fancy house.

If you know that you don't have separation please don't skip over this section – your abdominals have been stretched during your pregnancy and there is still much value in going through and learning what I am about to cover. You are still rebuilding strength and endurance, and knowing the potential warning signs, so that you can look out for yourself or educate other mums returning to exercise, is all part of your journey and adds to the support you can offer others.

Exercise: Push-ups

How to recognise a weakness:

Peaking or protruding of the abdominal wall resulting in a pyramid-type bulge that is visible and sticks out between the two sides of your rectus abdominals.

Quick check:

- You will need to be in front of a mirror (or place a mirror below you), or ask your partner or a friend to help you check your abdominals
- Start by doing a push-up on your knees; make sure you have the correct set-up and alignment, with your hands directly beneath your shoulders
- If you have a friend to help, ask them to put their hand across your abdominals and to hold it there
- If they feel a peak even before you begin the exercise then this position alone is too difficult for you right now and you need to make it easier
- If your tummy is relatively flat in your start position you should lower down towards the ground and ask for feedback from your friend – does this change and result in a peak as the position gets harder, or does it stay the same and you can maintain control?

How to love your body as much as your baby

- If your tummy peaks as you lower down you should make your push-up easier as this is too strong an exercise for you at this time
- If you don't have a friend to help, use your mirror and look for a change in the appearance of your abdominals, and for the telltale peaking

What to do:

- Decrease intensity by placing your hands on a raised surface (i.e. a bench or step)
- Repeat the quick check above
- IF you CAN – now lower into your push-up without any peaking, you can continue at this level
- IF you CAN'T – continue to make your push-up easier by raising your hands further, or by reducing the range of motion (or depth) of your push-up
- Ask for feedback from your friend at these different levels, to monitor and work out the best intensity for you at this time

Exercise: Prone hold

As mentioned in our pelvic floor section, many people think that a prone position is the perfect exercise to build strength through your core. But a prone creates a considerable amount of intra-abdominal pressure, which will push out through a weakened pelvic floor and abdominal wall – it should not be used as your go-to exercise for building core strength. Make sure you complete your rebuilding exercises prior to getting to this one.

How to recognise a weakness:

Peaking or protruding of the abdominal wall resulting in a pyramid-type bulge that is visible and sticks out between the two sides of your rectus abdominals.

Quick check:

- You will need to be in front of a mirror (or place a mirror below you), or ask your partner or a friend to help you check your abdominals
- Start by doing your prone on your knees, make sure you have the correct set-up and alignment, with your shoulders over your elbows
- If you have a friend to help, ask them to put their hand across your abdominals and to hold it there
- If they feel a peak, even when you are in your prone position, this exercise is too difficult for you right now and you need to make it easier
- If your tummy is relatively flat in this position you may hold here for longer. As you hold, ask your friend for feedback as to whether the tone in your abdominal wall changes. If, as you fatigue, a peak is felt, you should come down and work to this level for the time being

- If your tummy peaks immediately you should move back to a four-point position as a prone is too strong an exercise for you at this time
- If you don't have a friend to help, use your mirror and look for a change in the appearance of your abdominals and for the telltale peaking

What to do:

- Decrease intensity by moving straight away into an all-fours position with your hands directly beneath your shoulders and your knees directly beneath your hips
- Most women should be able to at least work at decreasing their peaking in this position using our abdominal breathing and TA activation exercise

I have used these two exercises as examples as they are the most obvious and because gravity adds pressure to your abdominal wall when performing them.

You will find that if you carry out these checks throughout every exercise in your workouts you will discover the telltale peaking during some of them. This will add pressure and potentially push your rectus abdominals apart (or at least prevent them coming together). I have seen a significant peaking, even during a triceps push-down, which would have thought would be a reasonably safe postnatal exercise. My answer to this is that yes, the exercise itself may be considered a safe one, but if the intensity is too high, or the exercise is not performed well, then the additional intra-abdominal pressure it creates means that your inner unit is not yet able to cope.

The key thing throughout your journey is to try not to become disheartened. It would have been easy to just carry on ignoring all of the signs that your body needs some extra help and just power on through towards your goal. I understand that it can be a little frustrating when you are forced to slow down for a while.

The main thing I say to all of the mums that I work with, and I say the same to you, is that this is your journey and you should feel empowered now that you know exactly what is going on with your body both inside and out. Your body has done an amazing thing in giving birth to your baby. It is now time for you to nurture it and build it back up in the safest and most efficient way. What I am giving you is the know-how to do this. Commit to your journey and with time and patience you will get there.

Real Mums

Sally, mother to Sophie (20m)

Having a baby has been the most amazing experience of my life. But nobody tells you how hard it can also be.

I was such an energetic kid, really fit and active, and I played lots of sports. Then puberty hit (I think my boobs threw out my balance or something) and my super fitness slowly crept into self-consciousness, and times of awesome laziness. I have been on quite a rollercoaster with my body, with some fitness and weight fluctuations over the years. I liked to blame it on genetics, but I'm sure the couch and a few packets of Tim Tams also came into play.

Falling pregnant had its challenges with Polycystic Ovary Syndrome (PCOS), but after a few years…success! The first six weeks were bliss and I was very excited, then the horrendous nausea and vomiting started. I kept trying to eat, as that would help with the nausea, but the volume of carbs I consumed far exceeded what was bouncing back out again! So the weight gain during pregnancy got off to a flying start.

The final three months I also had polyhydramnios, which is excessive amniotic fluid. They couldn't find a cause, but this excess fluid can cause pressure and restriction of blood flow to the baby so I had to be pretty closely monitored.

Exercise in that last few months was not possible, and I was the size of a whale! Once or twice they thought they would have to deliver the baby early, however I managed to carry to term. On 9 August 2011, after thirty-plus hours of labour (ouch), and finally an emergency caesarean, our beautiful, healthy baby girl was born.

It's amazing how quickly you fall in love with these new little creatures. Life is beautiful, but hard work too. I could write my own book about all the things I experienced in the first few months, but will highlight just a few:

- Inability to breastfeed = guilt
- Continuing attempts to breastfeed but failing = guilt
- Exclusively expressing breast milk for months = guilt
- Continuous sleep deprivation and crankiness = guilt
- Sophie getting reflux with nights of screaming and arching in pain, unable to feed and losing weight, with me crying unable to make her pain go away = guilt
- And, constant sleep deprivation!!!!

Did I mention enough guilt in there?

I have always felt I was very strong and resilient, and felt I was coping pretty damn well with each of these hurdles as they occurred. The thing about depression and anxiety, though, is that it sometimes sneaks up on you. It wasn't until Sophie was about six months old, and just starting that lovely period called 'separation anxiety', that I realised something more than just tiredness and a slightly emotional Mummy was occurring. Every time I walked away I deeply *felt* her tears, her fear and distress. My heart ached for her. I fiercely wanted to protect her from feeling hurt, from feeling pain, and feeling fear. I was increasingly anxious about my impending return to work date and leaving her. I loved my girl so much, overwhelmingly so. But with all the effort and focus on her, I was slowly starting to feel like I was losing myself, my identity. Sometimes I even felt a teeny bit trapped. Deep down I knew I needed to do some things for myself. One day, I found myself so tired and irrationally teary that I finally saw my wonderful GP who arranged blood tests and sent me to a psychologist.

Blood tests showed I had Hashimoto's Disease, where I have squillions of antibodies attacking my thyroid. This is another condition which can sometimes affect postnatal women, and also contributes to depression. Down the track, this eventually led to hypothyroidism for me, and it's now controlled with thyroxine.

The psychologist I saw was okay, but encouraged a huge number of natural supplements, which I wasn't super keen on. I would have tried another psychologist, but then I found Body Beyond Baby!

When I arrived for my first session in the park, I felt a little self-conscious. I was still very overweight and my exercise to that point had only been occasional walking. I had had very little time away from Sophie because I felt guilty leaving her. Most of all, I was really worried about Sophie crying for the nannies who were to look after her while I exercised. This sounds so silly, but by this stage I was so tired and emotional, that I was anxious about becoming more anxious!

Of course, the nannies were amazing, so friendly and understanding. And yes, Sophie did cry and I had to go and attend to her, but that was the stage she was going through. Little did I know that this was actually a form of therapy for me and Sophie – I was learning to leave her and know she would be okay. Slowly my guilty feelings ebbed and I could feel okay about mummy time. And of course, Sophie was learning that Mummy can walk away, but she always comes back, and much happier than before!

When I started training with Jen that first day, I was surprised at how out of condition I was. I struggled to make it around the oval, and had to start gently. I learned about my pelvic floor, and about abdominal separation, exercises to help my body repair, and those to avoid. Thank goodness I came to Body Beyond Baby, otherwise I would have been ab crunching in vain for years, wondering why I wasn't healing! I felt super unfit compared to the other mums but that comparison was only in my head. All of these women had started somewhere, all had their stories and they all had their weaknesses to work on. I loved coming to sessions and talking with these ladies, forming amazing friendships and feeling stronger and happier within myself.

One of the best things about starting training with Body Beyond Baby was doing the initial testing. Even today, whenever a new challenge starts, I love learning where my fitness levels are at and seeing how they improve over time. Measuring with the scales, tape measures and callipers tells me about my body shape and size (but there is no better test than how

How to love your body as much as your baby

my skinny jeans fit!), and then I hit the park for timed runs (or walks), beep tests, push-ups and strength tests that tell me where I'm at.

By getting a starting point, you can set yourself some goals, goals that are important to YOU. And what I found was that my goals really inspired my journey to fitness! Having a target to aim towards keeps up the excitement and momentum. Smashing those targets you set and going further gives you a sense of achievement and pride. You are not competing against the other mums, you are doing this for yourself.

And the scariest bit of initially starting was also the best – a 'before' shot. Yes, it is scary to lift the shirt and take a photo, but it is so amazing to SEE the results, simply awesome.

Going through this process with a group of amazing women, all on their own personal journey to fitness, has been wonderful. It is great hearing about, and seeing, everyone's achievements. And also having support there on the days you find it tough.

Training outdoors for me is fantastic; it's so good for the soul. When it rains, I feel like I've accomplished even more! Variety is so important, and doing a combination of cardio and resistance training is key, especially interval training (such great results for overall fitness!). My body achieved good strong foundations, and I have continued to build on that. I have a great personal trainer who sees my potential and pushes me to even more amazing results.

While the first six months of my daughter's life were spent running away from the camera from embarrassment, now I am happily in photos, and am even able to wear a bikini on the beach with confidence.

My journey of postnatal fitness has been life changing. Physically, I am fitter, leaner, stronger than ever before. I have achieved great results and want to continue to improve. Physical activity is part of my everyday life, I just move more! I get outdoors and have fun. And this is the best thing for Sophie too.

Mentally, I am happier and more resilient than ever. There is no depression. There is no anxiety. I love to exercise, and have felt firsthand the benefits it has on your overall health and wellbeing.

It is hard, as a mum, to find the time, but you have to. It is as important as any appointment you schedule. Be creative. Find the time. When your little monkey is asleep, hit the lounge room floor for some resistance band exercises, do some cardio, or try some high intensity interval training. Or even better, get Daddy to mind your little one after work while you disappear for an hour!

The future is so bright. I love it!

Gina, mother to Amélie (8m)

My Body Beyond Baby journey started eight weeks after I gave birth to my beautiful baby girl (now eight and a half months). I didn't really exercise before or during pregnancy and as a result I put on about 25 kilos, which certainly did not make me feel good about myself.

The first few training sessions were tough: I was overweight, struggled with technique, came last at everything and had a new born baby to look after. Luckily, I was surrounded by super-fit mums and fantastic trainers who encouraged and inspired me to take the next step and join the Body Beyond Baby Find Your Summer Body – 8 Week Challenge.

The beginning of the challenge involved recording my various body measurements and weight, photos were taken, and I completed the beep test and cardio test to the best of my ability. This was very uncomfortable for me but it was important to understand my starting point. It was then time to think about setting specific goals that were measurable and attainable in the eight-week period: my main goal was to lose six kilos.

I hadn't really been doing any pelvic floor exercises and didn't really know if I was doing them properly so Jen recommended a pelvic floor workshop held by women's health physiotherapist, Jo Murdoch. There I explained that when I ran I felt a heavy feeling which was something I had not felt before. With Real Time Ultrasound it became evident that I had a very weak pelvic floor so I was given specific pelvic floor rebuilding exercises to do every day for the next six weeks. I was also advised not to run (walking only), to undertake every exercise at the easiest level (which meant push-ups and prone holds were to be completed on my knees) and to and use the lowest strength elastic for resistance training. I was taught, and learned how, to adapt each exercise to train to my weakest link.

Over the next six weeks I exercised as per the advice I'd been given and religiously completed my rebuilding exercises. When I visited Jo again I learned that my pelvic floor had improved by 50 percent. New pelvic floor exercises were provided and I was given the go ahead to start running and increase my level of training.

At the end of the eight weeks I felt fantastic! I'd lost weight and changed my body shape, and I felt fitter, stronger and much happier than I had in a long time. This came at a great time for me as I was heading home to the UK for an extended trip over Christmas and the New Year. I returned for the beginning of the next challenge and I couldn't wait to get started. With my new found fitness and strength I was able to step up my training, increase the elastic strength used when completing resistance training and…fit into my pre-pregnancy jeans comfortably!

I recently had a third pelvic floor check-up and was pleased to learn that I now have a strong pelvic floor – I was told to 'go for my life' in terms of exercise. I truly believe in the importance of rebuilding from the inside out, exercising using the correct technique, good nutrition and being part of a great community of mums who support and inspire each other. Body Beyond Baby has provided me with the tools to lose weight, gain strength, get fitter and feel fantastic so I can be the best mum I can be for my daughter.

5 Easy To Implement Actions

1. Do a variety of cardio and resistance exercise

2. Choose interval training for cardio, and compound exercises for resistance

3. Remember to keep challenging yourself – as your body gets stronger and fitter you will need to make your workout harder to keep seeing results

4. Rest is important too

5. Know your limitations and train to your current weakest link

Nurture from the Inside Out

Nutrition plays a huge role in our health and wellness. Many of our habits were learned a long time ago when we were children and where we are today, in terms of what we eat, is part of the journey that is unique to each of us. Our nutrition, just like our exercise is tweaked and changed as we go. As we learn, we implement new or healthier ways to eat.

If you look at my diet now you might think it's quite extreme. I read an article recently about a celebrity chef who completely overhauled his diet. The feedback from his readers was exactly that, that his diet was extreme or unrealistic but for me what he was eating for breakfast was very normal and not too dissimilar to my own diet, today. But had you looked at my diet eight to 10 years ago, it would have been a different story.

Wherever you are on your journey, there is no right or wrong. We all come from different places, have been brought up in different ways, and some of us have more or less to learn than others. It is easy to look at me and assume I have always eaten in the way that I do now, and that it's just easy. Yes, it is easy but it has been a journey – a long one.

Nutrition is a journey

My Story

I was brought up with two influences. My mum and dad divorced when I was quite young which meant my sister and I lived at both Mum's house and Dad's house. From the outside it may have looked like a confusing and hard-to-keep-track-of arrangement but for us spending every Monday, Wednesday and every other Friday, Saturday and Sunday at Dad's house, and every Tuesday, Thursday and every other Friday, Saturday and Sunday at Mum's house, somehow worked. We had two ways of many things: a shared bedroom or our own rooms, TV allowed in our rooms in one house but not in the other. These two ways also included two ways of eating.

I also had my own theories and ideas. At 12-years old I decided I was going to become vegetarian. And what started as a new thing to try with a classmate turned into 14-years of not eating meat. I started off eating fish but after a traumatic experience with swordfish (which for a non-meat eater was like eating a huge piece of white steak) I decided fish was off the menu too.

How to love your body as much as your baby

There was always healthy food in the fridge at Mum's house and she continued to put healthy food on the table, and so did Dad. As I got older, however, I became more and more fussy when it came to vegetables; I didn't like broccoli or cauliflower or sprouts, actually I didn't particularly care for many veggies at all. At a certain point Dad got bored with experimenting with meals that I constantly rejected so I was left to feed myself when staying at his place. I thought this was fantastic; we could go food shopping with him and put whatever we wanted into the trolley.

I ate a lot of microwaved meals and pot noodles over the years that followed and I also established my love of pasta. In fact, pasta became my staple diet – for a vegetarian who didn't eat vegetables there wasn't a lot else on offer. But I was happy. My favourite meal became a pasta bake type concoction: pasta and tomato sauce (no added veggies) with sliced boiled potatoes and cheese on top. I carried this meal with me for years and when I left England and came to Australia at 18 it was still a regular feature on my weekly menu.

Throughout this time I was eating lots of sugar too. At Mum's house there was little sugar in the house. We might have the odd biscuit if we were lucky, but there certainly were never any packets of chips or chocolate bars floating around, no cakes or lollies or junk food in general. At Dad's though, my sister and I could choose sugary snacks and chips; we thought it was great. As I got older, and I learned to drive, my friends and I would regularly go to the McDonald's drive-through and eat Happy Meals; my car back window was once covered in their free toys. I realise now I was a great advertisement for Happy Meals – certainly not the advertisement I strive to be now!

In terms of exercise, I competed in gymnastics until the age of 14 and then, although still training a little, I slowed down. You can get away with eating rubbish for a while but eventually the reduced movement and the awful fuel you are putting into your body catches up with you. By the time I had been in Australia for about six months, at age 18, living on my diet of pasta, potatoes and cheese (and the bowl of ice cream with Ice Magic that I had taken up for dessert most evenings) I was tipping the scales at a less than healthy weight for me, which was most definitely not made up of heavier muscle mass.

Slowly, but surely, I began to take note of what I was doing and something clicked within me. Whether it was the idea of donning a bikini on the beach in summertime, or the good foundations that had been laid for me when I was small, I decided it was time to get myself together, make some changes and get healthy again.

I find that between 18 and our early 20s many of us lose our way. No matter what our parents have taught us, we generally eat more rubbish –because no one is telling us not to, and move less – because we are no longer at school and often haven't discovered the gym yet. We prefer to spend our time with friends, eating out, drinking and enjoying life, thinking that we are still young and can still eat junk to the same extent as when we were burning it off twice as fast.

It is when we stop and take note that we can begin to go back to what we know we should be eating, if, and only if, we have been taught this to begin with.

Why Great Foundations are so Important

I have a client who is twenty-eight; she is not yet a mother but looks after children as part of her work. She tells me stories of never, ever being given vegetables as a child. Her mother would try her with a new food and if she spat it out would just assume she didn't like it and wouldn't bother again, not through lack of caring but because she, herself didn't have the education to know to keep trying. When I met her she had an extremely limited diet – McDonald's and pizzas, chips and chocolate were pretty much what her diet consisted of on a daily basis. She didn't like to eat vegetables and there was a huge number of foods that she either didn't like or had never tried. Imagine at twenty-eight not ever having eaten salmon before, not liking tomatoes, and living on junk foods.

She has now come a long way. She has read a lot and worked with me, and together we are on a journey to help her form new eating patterns, but it is hard. Undoing almost every habit you have around food is a hard thing to do and I see the battles she has. I also see her passion to ensure the same thing doesn't happen to the children she cares for. I hear her stories of their parents leaving lunch boxes containing Freddo Frogs,

Vegemite sandwiches, chips and juice; she will now go out and buy them chicken and fruit and healthy foods instead. She is well read on the topic of nutrition, and is even considering studying, but the foundations that were laid for her as a child prove a constant barrier to her making a new, healthier way of life that feels like it comes naturally.

I am very lucky that despite the different tracks I have taken with food and nutrition I had a good, solid foundation given to me when I was small. I now eat in a way, and teach my children to eat in a way, that might even make what I ate then look unhealthy now. But it is those good food foundations that have made it easier for me to come full circle and continue my journey to here.

No matter where you are on your journey, and no matter what your foundations, you can use the knowledge you will learn in this book to benefit both yourself and your children. You can lay the tracks ahead – if you were given great foundations as a child you can build upon them, and if you weren't you can start to lay your own foundations.

Whatever your story, I do know that the education you undertake yourself is vital to what you will pass down to the next generation. Educate yourself well and pass that on to your children, lay their foundations and set them up to live the healthiest life they can. They may stray along the way, and they more than likely will as they take the reins as they grow. But, I believe that if you teach them well they will eventually come back to what they know and make decisions to change whatever they need to, to eat healthily and well – just like you are doing now.

How to love your body as much as your baby

Tried and Tested

The nutritional information I provide in this book has been tried and tested by over 250 mums who have been part of the winter and summer challenges within my business, Body Beyond Baby. When these have been combined with their commitment to exercise and taking time out for themselves they have seen some absolutely fantastic results. Mums have lost body fat, centimetres and have reported increased levels of energy. Others, as a result of their own education and transformation, have turned around the diet of their whole household and are now feeding everyone much cleaner and healthier options.

Simple and Sustainable

The information given here is designed to offer you a guide on how to make some simple and sustainable changes to your way of eating. It will not tell you *exactly* what to eat, and it will not give you whole and complete menu plans, as I truly believe that specific eating plans do not teach you well about how to choose the best nutrition for yourself and your family.

Yes, it would be very easy to just follow a plan. But, given that no one plan would suit everybody, and that my aim is to provide you with information that will lead to long-term change, I will do things differently than many exercise and fitness books. I am here to give you the tools, and for you to take responsibility for the job at hand. I can't feed you and I am not willing to leave you without the ability to eat well once your program has finished. I believe there is too much of an on/off mentality when we embark upon an eating plan. When you make the decision to make changes to your health and wellbeing you need to do so at your own pace.

You might have a brand new baby and, for you, following an eating plan is just not on the cards right now. What you need to do is take a few simple steps towards making changes at your own pace and, when you are ready, take a few more. You may be further down the track and ready to completely overhaul your nutritional intake, in which case you may be able to absorb every scrap of information in this book and run with it.

What I will say to everyone, regardless of where you are at and how old your children are, is that you need to implement things that you can commit to for the long-term. If something feels extreme it probably is. If it is too far from what you are doing right now you may find it hard to sustain for the long haul and the last thing you want to do is fall into a cycle of all or nothing. When you look back in a year's time you may very well have completely overhauled your diet and implemented everything in this book, but for now you must take steps day by day. Make little changes and reap the rewards of working towards a healthier you both inside and out.

> **Take simple steps day by day**

How to love your body as much as your baby

As we move forward, you will learn how to make healthier choices for you and your family. Some things will be reminders of information you may already know and need to tune into once again. I have also included lots of additional information that you need to be aware of to achieve your personal goals. What you put into your mouth will contribute greatly to how successful you are in your quest for YOUR best ever body.

If you choose not to alter your food intake at all, and not to make these healthier changes, you will have to train so much harder to see the results you might wish. And it is true; you cannot out-train a bad diet.

Remember that you have made the choice to learn how to love YOUR body and how to discover YOUR best ever body; to change your lifestyle so you can feel fantastic from the inside out. Eating well is essential to a happy and healthy you.

Benefits of a Healthy Diet

- Increased energy levels and vitality
- Lower risk of disease, such as heart disease or Type 2 Diabetes
- Control over your bodyweight
- Increased sense of wellbeing
- Better self-esteem and body image
- Better concentration
- Stronger bones and teeth

To improve your diet and ensure you are making the best possible food choices use this guide on a day-to-day basis;

- Preparation and consistency are the key
- Begin your day with a good healthy breakfast
- Stop eating while you are still comfortable; it's okay to leave food on your plate
- Allow your body to register that it has eaten, wait for an hour – if you are still hungry reach for a healthy snack
- Carry healthy snacks with you
- Include a protein source in every meal or snack
- Reach for low GI carbohydrates
- Read labels – check the sugar content as well as the fat content, and if you can't read it, don't eat it!
- Eat a wide variety of coloured fruit and veggies
- Eat every few hours to ensure your metabolism keeps burning
- Enjoy smaller meals of an evening
- Eat at least two hours before going to bed
- Drink plenty of water, especially when exercising

How to love your body as much as your baby

The Law of Energy Balance:

To lose weight, you must burn more calories than you consume each day

To gain weight, you must consume more calories than you burn each day

Never Skip Meals

Skipping meals (or leaving long gaps between meals) is one of the worst things you can do when your goal is fat loss while maintaining muscle mass (and we want to maintain muscle mass to maintain your metabolic rate).

Missing meals slows down your metabolism and causes muscle loss. This then puts your body into starvation mode meaning that whatever you eat next will store as fat in preparation for the next time you starve it. You then skip another meal or two and the vicious cycle continues. You can see why you then struggle to lose body fat and potentially put on more weight in the long run.

Missing meals is a huge problem that I see particularly with mums. We are often swept up in looking after everyone else and our own nutritional needs take that back burner.

How many of us can relate to having got up, changed the baby, fed the baby, rocked the baby, taken the baby out because they were unsettled, grabbed a coffee as we sped past the coffee shop, took the baby home, fed the baby again, put the baby to bed, then realised its 1pm and we haven't had breakfast yet?!

Or you might be the mother of older children who has gotten up before them to have your own shower and get dressed, put their breakfast on the table, made a cup of tea and eaten a few spoonful's of their breakfast or yoghurt out of the tub while dishing up, hurried them to the table, encouraged eating, cleared the table, supervised getting dressed, negotiated TV time, packed bags, asked for shoes to be put on a hundred times, raced everyone out of the door and finally dropped them off at school and kindy at 8.58am only to realise you forgot your own breakfast, but now you have to rush to work or do the household chores with only time to grab a takeaway coffee and a sugar-loaded muffin on the way.

Always eat breakfast

If I can do no other thing apart from ensure that from now on you don't miss a meal – most specifically breakfast – I will be happy. When you are putting energy and love into doing the best possible thing for your child it is important that you are fuelled for your day and have put energy and love into yourself.

A Calorie is Not Just a Calorie

Although I don't recommend you start calorie counting, I do think it is great to have some knowledge in this area to help with your food choices.

Quick Calorie Information

A healthy diet is about good nutrition regularly throughout the day. This means we want to eat a variety of complex carbohydrates, lean proteins and healthy fats which will keep blood sugar levels stable and keep you satisfied.

	Calories Per Gram
Carbohydrates	4
Protein	4
Fat	9
Alcohol	7

Take note that fats and alcohol have double the amount of calories that carbohydrates and protein do.

A common obstacle in our quest for fat loss is the view that a calorie is just a calorie and all that matters is calories in, versus calories out. If it were as simple as that, then you could eat anything you wanted and you would still lose body fat, as long as your calories were in deficit. You could eat nothing but chocolate and drink just coke, and if you were 100 calories under maintenance level you would lose weight. We know that this is not true.

If a calorie is just a calorie, then three diets at the same calorie level, the first composed of 100 percent protein, the second 100 percent carbohydrates and the third 100 percent fats, would all have the same effect on body composition. I am sure you can imagine that a diet consisting of 100 percent chicken (lean protein) will not have the same effect as a diet consisting of 100 percent chips (fat and carbohydrate).

Avoid empty calories

In my opinion, all alcohol and refined sugar calories are empty calories – this means that they are of no nutritional value at all. In essence, you would be wasting your daily calories by consuming them, and depriving your body of valuable nutrients.

It is important to always combine a lean protein, complex carbohydrate food, and good fat, at every meal. By combining these nutrients you help to control the hormones responsible for fat storage and provide a steady flow of amino acids from protein foods for muscle growth and maintenance.

Pregnant and Breastfeeding Women

Pregnant women should not be aiming to lose weight unless specifically advised to by their doctor for the wellbeing of themselves and their baby. Instead, you should be concentrating on eating a balanced and healthy diet for you and your baby. Normal weight women should increase their ENERGY IN by approximately 300 healthy calories per day in their second and third trimester.

Breastfeeding women with a baby under six months old should continue to consume an additional 200 to 300 healthy calories per day to maintain a sufficient, nutritional milk supply.

Women with established breastfeeding babies are safely able to lose weight, so long as you maintain a nutritionally sound diet – if you starve yourself of vital nutrients your body has a clever way of giving those nutrients to your baby, leaving you depleted. Ensure you monitor your milk supply and your baby's reaction to a change in diet. Should you see a difference in the way they are feeding, adjust your calories and exercise accordingly.

It is also extremely important for all breastfeeding women to drink plenty of water to maintain hydration.

Portion Sizes

Portion sizes are one of the most important things to understand when monitoring ENERGY IN. Most of us need to learn to eat smaller meals, more often, to keep our metabolisms going.

To give you an idea:

- 150g of meat is about the size of the palm of your hand

- A serving of complex carbohydrates from starches or grains is the amount you can hold in a single cupped hand
- A serving of vegetables is what you can hold in two hands cupped together

Sugar

For many years we were told fat was bad and that we should eat low-fat everything. The trouble with this is that many low-fat foods have additional sugar and additives to make them taste good. And if low-fat is good for you, and most of our population is living by the low-fat craze, then why is it that we have a growing obesity epidemic?

Sugar comes in many forms and is included in many pre-packaged foods and sauces. I encourage you to be as vigilant as possible in avoiding sugar in all its forms.

Here is a list of hidden sugars – now you know that all of these words translate into sugar:

Agave nectar	Cane crystals
Barbados sugar	Cane juice crystals
Barley Malt	Cane sugar
Beet Sugar	Caramel
Blackstrap molasses	Carob syrup
Brown sugar	Castor sugar
Buttered syrup	Confectioner's sugar

Corn syrup	Honey
Corn sweetener	Icing sugar
Corn syrup solids	Invert sugar
Crystalline fructose	Lactose
Date sugar	Malt syrup
Demerara Sugar	Maltodextrin
Dextrin	Maltose
Dextran	Mannitol
Diastic malt	Maple syrup
Diastase	Molasses
D-mannose	Muscovado sugar
Evaporated cain juice	Organic raw sugar
Ethyl maltol	Panocha
Florida crystals	Powdered sugar
Florida crystals	Raw sugar
Fructose	Refiner's syrup
Fruit juice	Rice syrup
Fruit juice concentrate	Sorbitol
Galactose	Sorghum syrup
Glucose	Sucrose
Golden sugar	Sugar
Golden syrup	Syrup
Granulated sugar	Table sugar
Grape juice concentrate	Treacle
Grape sugar	Turbinado sugar
High-fructose corn syrup	Yellow sugar

I also recommend you avoid the following foods and beverages:

- Alcohol
- Cakes, chocolates, pastries, ice cream, lollies or soft drink
- Fruit juices, milkshakes or store-bought smoothies and juices
- White potato or white rice (this includes sushi)
- Sweetened yoghurt
- Sugar, including in tea or coffee
- Dried fruit (two to three pieces of fruit per day only is recommended)

All of these foods have little or no nutritional value at all and really just help to top up your diet with empty calories, calories that could be spent much more wisely on healthy, whole food alternatives.

Food on the Run

Snacks

Mums are often on the run so I have put together a list of foods that you can easily grab, most of which you can throw in your baby bag alongside your child's food to ensure you never get caught out needing that sugar-loaded muffin with your coffee.

How to love your body as much as your baby

- Veggie sticks – including carrot, celery, capsicum or snow peas – with hummus
- Medium piece of fruit and a small handful of nuts
- Plain yoghurt
- Cottage cheese and berries
- Hardboiled egg
- Tin of tuna in spring water
- 100 grams lean ham/chicken
- Smoked salmon, cream cheese and cucumber slices

Meals

You may think I am super prepared and always have my meals with me. Admittedly, I do always leave the house with my breakfast in a cool bag, along with snacks for my day as per the list above, but I am certainly not organised enough to make sure I have every meal with me also. I eat between one and three meals per day out of a food court or from a take away venue. I do, however, manage to eat very healthily and I'd like to share with you my food choices so that eating out can never again be an excuse for a poor diet.

- Choose Thai stir-fries either with no rice, or brown rice if this is an option
- Sashimi or brown rice sushi
- Grilled fish and salad
- Grilled chicken salad
- Bun-less burgers from burger places – yes, a lot of them will give you the meat and the salad without the bun!

Nurture from the Inside Out

- Poached egg, tomatoes, spinach, mushrooms, avocado and wholemeal sourdough
- Mexican bean salad or chicken salad

Occasional Foods

Although I have talked about avoiding sugar completely, I am well aware we all like to enjoy the sweeter things in life from time to time. For some, the odd sweet treat can easily be eaten, put down, and not thought about again. For others, a side step from a healthy eating plan can mean a slippery slide back to old habits. Given this is such an individual thing; I have chosen not to set specific occasional foods guidelines, but to let you decide what will work best for you.

The ideal scenario is that you commit to the foods to avoid and remove as much sugar from your life as possible. However, I take on board that special occasions arise and life doesn't always pan out that way. My aim is to enable you to live with your new eating and exercise patterns for the long-term. Therefore, you now need to decide what will be the best strategy for you. I encourage you to write it down and stick to it.

Keep a Food Diary

I have found one of the best and most effective ways of becoming accountable for, and aware of, what you are putting into your mouth is to start writing it down. This doesn't have to go on forever, but many of the mums I work with are absolutely amazed when they compare what they think they are eating on a daily basis and what they are actually eating. The extra muffin they grabbed as a one-off (which is more like every day); finishing off their children's meals every night before their own dinner; the one or two treats which somehow blow easily out of control and become a regular fixture. Your food diary is especially helpful when you are trying to out-train a diet that has sometimes gone off the rails during pregnancy.

It's also a great way to look at the balance in your diet. Are you living on pasta and carbohydrates? Are the good fats missing from your diet? Do you eat too much or too little protein?

Make the commitment to write it down for a week, or at least three days, without making any conscious changes and then start to refine and change a few things each week as you go. When you do this and keep documenting your eating it's really cool to see your progression – where you have come from and what you have achieved in cleaning up your diet.

Introducing Belinda Kirkpartick

I have worked in partnership with Belinda for over three years in developing the nutritional elements of Body Beyond Baby. My clients always find her information valuable and informative and we continue to see fantastic results within our programs.

Belinda is a university-qualified nutritionist and naturopath and mummy of two gorgeous girls. She has been in clinical practice for over eight years and has helped hundreds of women and their families reach their optimal health potential.

Belinda specialises in women's health, preconception (including fertility management and miscarriage reduction), pregnancy, postnatal care, babies' and children's health. Belinda continues to research and study extensively, she holds a Bachelor of Health Science (Naturopathy), an Associate Degree in Clinical Sciences, an Advanced Diploma of Naturopathy and is currently completing a Masters of Reproductive Medicine in the School of Women's and Children's Health at the University of New South Wales.

Belinda's Top 5 Expert Tips to Nurturing the Body From the Inside Out

1. **Eat whole foods.** Whole foods are close to nature and give nutrition and energy that cannot be replicated in a factory.

2. **Sugar really is the enemy.** Avoid it at all costs (and watch your cravings and your waistline reduce). Check the ingredients in all processed foods you buy (crackers, muesli, yoghurt etc.) and stop buying products with added sugars.

3. Be realistic. Which are your every day foods and which are your sometimes foods? Being healthy is not about being perfect all the time. If 90 percent of your diet is good, it is fine to eat an unhealthy food (without guilt) from time to time, BUT be honest with yourself. If you eat a biscuit, a little chocolate or some banana bread several days a week, it is now no longer just a sometimes food for you or your children and therefore not great for your health!

4. Be mindful of your digestive system. Bloating, gas and irregular bowel movements are signs you are not absorbing all the nutrients in your food.

5. Make time to relax and breathe every day. Even as mums, we can all make time twice a day to take ten slow, deep, nourishing belly breaths. Your body (and mind) will thank you.

More from Belinda

In pregnancy, most women are very aware of eating healthy foods and the impact these foods will have on their growing baby. After pregnancy, many women abandon these eating principles and return to eating a high-carbohydrate, low-nutrient, comfort food diet. I cannot stress enough the importance of continuing healthy eating after your baby is born. The same healthy food you ate during pregnancy will support your own body to maintain health, energy and happiness throughout life.

You are important – as a mother and as a unique and special woman. Acknowledge this, by making enough time to plan, create and eat simple, healthy meals. Many new mums I work with tell me they are so busy looking after their baby and/or other children they do not have time to eat breakfast, plan snacks or sit down and eat lunch each day themselves! If you stock your fridge and cupboards with processed, unhealthy and nutritionally deficient, convenience foods, that is what you (and your family) will eat. Making a conscious decision to stock up on healthy whole foods means even on your craziest days at home, your choices will have to be good. It also means your children will not whinge and whine until you give them that packet of chips, the sweet biscuit or the lolly they are begging for. When they know it isn't there, your job is so much easier!

Many young babies will eat lots of different vegetables, fruits, proteins, legumes and natural yoghurts. However, by the time they are two- or three-years of age, many parents report their children have become fussy and less willing to eat the foods they once enjoyed. Their range of foods becomes narrower and narrower. Why is this? Are you modelling healthy eating by sitting down to regular meals; snacking on vegetables, hummus or nuts; experimenting with different foods and flavours? For many, the answer is no. Most mums tell me they want their children to be healthy and happy and to eat a wide variety of healthy foods, yet if we are not modelling good eating habits this way of eating is not seen as normal to our children. Unless they see you eating and enjoying the foods you want them to eat, you have little chance of convincing them to eat or enjoy them. Makes sense doesn't it? The reason little children in India eat dhal and curries, or Vietnamese children eat vegetable-laden pho soup, is not because they are different from our children, it's because they see their parents eating those foods on a regular basis and so it's normal for them. What is normal in your home? What would you like it to be?

Think about yourself and your role models. On the whole, women who find it natural to prioritise their health and fitness are often those who grew up in homes where their parents exercised regularly and ate healthy foods. Many women who grew up having sweet desserts after dinner every

How to love your body as much as your baby

night are among those who experience intense sugar cravings after meals and constantly struggle against this desire. Interestingly, many of them are also regularly giving their children dessert after dinner (flavoured yoghurts, ice-blocks, etc.), sometimes using these as an incentive to get them to eat their main meal, as if the main meal is something unpleasant to be endured to get the reward of an unhealthy sweet treat! What habits are you setting up for your children? A life of fighting against sweet cravings after meals, or one where the healthy main meal is satisfying and sufficient?

Healthy eating is not just about avoiding unhealthy foods, but choosing healthy foods which are nutritionally dense and which help your body to achieve optimal health. My clients will know exactly what I mean by not filling yourself and your little ones with shut-up foods. These foods fill up your stomach and stop you feeling hungry but, while they may not always be unhealthy, they give you little nutritional value in return. They include foods like dry crackers, commercial cereals, Vegemite or jam toast and plain pasta.

Do not underestimate the impact of making small changes. Although children brought up with healthy choices may be more open to eating quinoa, chia seeds and coconut smoothies, children brought up on less healthy foods can change over time – just don't try a full dietary overhaul in one day! If you can be patient and realistic about timeframes when working with children, showing them you are enjoying these new foods, they will begin to accept them slowly but surely. For fussy eaters, start with very small amounts of new foods, for an easy win. As the new foods begin to be accepted, you can slowly increase the amount and variety given. For an older child it may take months to completely change their diet, but the wait is worth it.

Nurture from the Inside Out

Real Mums

Jasmin, mother to Layla(2)

How it all started – being the big kid

I never remember being small. I was always the big kid – taller, heavier and older than my age. When I look back at my year-seven photo, having reached puberty early, I look like the teacher sitting in the front row. I was not a fat child but my weight battle has been ever-present. I remember wearing the same size clothes as my mum before I entered high school and saw this as a sign of maturity. My parents always ensured that we had a healthy and balanced diet. They did the best they could with what they knew. My downfall was always treat food. The problem was that every day there were treat foods. In my HSC year I would demolish a packet of lollies every night while studying, in an attempt to maintain concentration; at the end of the year, I rolled out of my study and cried too many tears when looking for a formal dress. I never played competitive sport, the monkey bars always eluded me, and I always preferred walking over running. My parents bought me my first gym membership at 15 and it was here that my journey with weight management began. I've been a regular exerciser from that time but my diet was what let me down, time and time again. Don't get me wrong – I thought I had a healthy, balanced diet. I rarely ate junk food, I didn't binge drink and I didn't skip meals (I loved food too much!).

My downfall was, and has always been, my love of sugar.

My journey so far – leaving an abusive relationship for a better life

Through my late teens and 20s, my weight yo-yoed between a size 14 and a size 18. There were bigger and smaller years but all in all, I was a bigger girl. I never wore a bikini or a midriff top. I accepted that this was how I was. I continued to exercise with little to any results. Before meeting my husband, I went on a massive exercise onslaught and lost 10 kilos to get down to 80 kilos, despite paying little to any attention to my diet. I was the lightest I remembered but felt that this weight was difficult to maintain. Sure enough, my weight crept back up until I was diagnosed as being insulin resistant. Through medication, a low GI diet, and exercise, I managed to once again return to 80 kilos before I got married. When I contemplated falling pregnant, I was petrified of getting gestational diabetes. Throughout my pregnancy, I watched what I ate and trained with a prenatal trainer. My regular blood tests returned normal readings, I only gained 10 kilos while pregnant and I managed to avoid gestational diabetes. Maternity leave, postnatal depression and an absence of exercise due to severe sleep deprivation saw me turn to food as comfort – I stacked on the weight thanks to eating all night when I breastfed and seeking to address my exhaustion with sugar. Even though my insulin resistance had abated, when I had to buy size 18 jeans to get out of track pants and found myself cutting out the tag, I realised that it was time for me to address

Nurture from the Inside Out

my weight gain, again. I re-started my training and lost some of the weight but my focus was primarily on exercise rather than diet.

I had trained with Body Beyond Baby sporadically for the months leading up to the 2012 'Watch Your Winter Waist Line Challenge' and I knew that this was an opportunity to turn things around. I was ready to make a change and jumped in with both feet. I aimed to lose six kilos and get back to my normal level. Apart from committing to training five to six times a week, I finally took charge of my diet. The challenge had a four-week sugar free period that involved removing all added sugar, potatoes and white rice and limiting the consumption of bread. Considering that this challenge was only 12 weeks, I figured that I had nothing to lose and went sugar free from day one! After four weeks, apart from losing four kilos, I noticed that my 20-year battle with scalp psoriasis had ended; no more scratching, flaking or pain. Could it be my diet? Could it be the removal of wheat?

I was overjoyed by my weight loss and the changes I saw. I kept my foot to the pedal and by the eight-week mark, I had lost nine kilos and passed level I was aiming for. I still had four weeks to go. It was at this point that Jen challenged me to consider trying grain free. At first I balked. No way. What would I eat? But when I looked at my diet, the only grains remaining were morning oats and the odd sandwich. From that point on I gave up grains and never looked back.

I feel so much better. No more bloating, I don't feel heavy after I eat, and I never feel hungry. By the end of the challenge

How to love your body as much as your baby

I had lost almost 12 kilos, double my original goal, and I was well below any weight I could remember being. Beyond the challenge, I have lost more weight and stayed sugar and grain free. This is not a diet but a lifestyle. I ended an abusive relationship I had with food. I used to give bad food all my love and attention. What I got back was abuse. Despite the effect the food had on me, I kept giving it my love. One day I woke up and realised that I had to get out of this abusive relationship. I packed my bag and never looked back!

Laying the right foundations from the start

So now I'm a mum. I have a little girl who looks to me for guidance on life. I have such a valuable opportunity to show her the right way to treat her body so that it gives her the most it has to offer. I am extremely conscious of my weight battle history and her genetic makeup from both my, and my husband's, sides of the family. Given my journey, I am confronted by the cultural norm that childhood equals sugar; it seems to be accepted that it's okay to eat heaps of sugar as a kid. I am determined to not let my daughter fall victim to the sugar trap that I once spent battling. I made a decision early on that sugar would not feature in her diet. I had plenty of push-back from family and friends as well as strangers, other parents and preschool. I am constantly made to feel like my attitudes and approach are strange, mean and restrictive. If my child was diabetic, no one would argue with my decision to restrict sugar in her diet. Why do people find this choice so strange? My daughter doesn't miss out. She has a varied diet. I cook for her every day and ensure that I regularly bake for her too. She has cake, ice cream and treats. The difference is that these foods are sugar free and healthy. She knows no different. There will come a time when I can no longer control her diet as I once did. I hope that by giving her the right start and by setting a good example, she will continue to honour her body, value the food she eats and realise the effect food has on the potential her body holds.

Where to from here?

I have made a lifestyle choice and I have no plan to ever go back. I need to exercise every day for my physical, mental and emotional wellbeing. Some may see my dietary choices as radical or overboard but they work for me and my family. I am healthier, lighter, happier and stronger than I have ever been. I don't ever again want to be that girl cutting out size labels from jeans to hide her weight. I know that I have inspired, and continue to inspire, many with the transformation I have made. Most of all, I want to be a role model for my daughter so she knows that hard work and dedication will bring amazing results.

I have always loved to cook and still do. Nowadays, I look to adapt recipes by removing sugar and grains. I substitute where I can and experiment often. I always make sure our meals are filling and interesting. I cook in advance and I plan our weekly meals. I take my food with me whenever I can and talk about lifestyle change whenever I get a chance. Overall, this has been a journey of reduction to elimination,

How to love your body as much as your baby

trial and error. Nothing has happened overnight. I have grown into this lifestyle and adapted it to suit me. My advice is to never be scared to give something a go. Trial it for a week. If you can't do without it, go back and reduce it week by week. Be honest and admit there are foods you struggle with. I have a sugar addiction. I can't eat one lolly; I need to eat the whole packet. As a result, I know I just can't start or tempt myself. Rather, I admit my addiction and steer clear. The food industry has done a fabulous job of convincing us of all the things we need in our diets. Stop, look, read and consider what's right for you and your family.

Della, mother to Milly(12), Rory(9), Henry(6) and Darcy(22m)

The family's eating habits

Before I embarked on my journey with Body Beyond Baby I was generally happy with my family's eating habits. We did not have a lot of junk food from fast food outlets and we all ate well balanced meals and snacks.

My active kids seem to be constantly hungry and sometimes, worn down by their whining, I would give in to their demands for snacks between meals, even before dinner. I gave them snacks which I considered to be relatively healthy, such as a peanut butter sandwich or a sweet biscuit (just one!), a tub of fruit yoghurt, or a whole piece of fruit.

As part of my efforts to watch their fat intake the whole family had light milk, and there were many other items in the

Nurture from the Inside Out

cupboard and the fridge which were labelled "lite", such as the margarine, the fruit yoghurt and the cheese. I knew that soft drink was not an everyday thing and I also knew that I should steer clear of fruit juice, which is filled with sugar. I knew that ice creams and chocolate bars were a special treat but sometimes I found that the treats were happening every few days rather than once a week.

What I did not know, however, was how much sugar is contained in other food that my kids were eating every day – the light yoghurt, the lashings of tomato sauce and mint sauce that accompanied every healthy meal, the healthy wholegrain breakfast cereal, the dried fruit, the little packet of Tiny Teddy's, the banana bread at the cafe or the healthy muesli bar that went in the lunch box every day.

It was when I started to look more carefully at my own consumption of sugar (and also grains) that I made some startling discoveries about what we had all been eating as a family. First of all I realised that my attempts to cut out fat were actually doing us all more harm than good – as all of the low-fat products I was buying often contained more sugar than the full-fat version. I also came to see that so much of what we were eating (even if it was light) was heavily processed and contained a number of different ingredients that were very surprising. I also worked out that I did not have to give the kids starchy carbohydrates such as bread, pasta or potato with every single meal.

I thought carefully about how to change my family's ways. I knew it might be a disaster if I suddenly cut out all the food that the kids were used to having, and replacing it with something new and less processed. I also needed to figure out what to give them and I was worried that it might take more time to feed them this way. I decided to start by making a few small changes and then to introduce more changes over time. I would do it by stealth!

The first change was an easy one – the family switched to full-fat A2 milk and full-fat Greek yoghurt. Breakfast was next – eggs and avocado was a real hit with nine-year old Rory. Surprisingly, once I bought a good non-stick pan, eggs became a quick and easy option. Porridge (with less and less sugar every time) also became a regular choice. There was no more sugary breakfast cereal left and I just somehow kept forgetting to buy any more!

The lunchboxes also went through a few changes as the weeks went by. No more little packets of biscuits. Instead there is seaweed, cottage cheese, boiled eggs, cherry tomatoes, plain popcorn or Greek yoghurt and fruit. I still throw in the occasional muesli bar but it is not an everyday thing as it once was. My family still has a way to go – I would love to see them devour a plate of vegie sticks and hummus – but we are moving in the right direction towards real, protein packed and fresh and away from shut-up food with no real nutritional value and heavily processed food.

The family's exercise habits

My husband and I place a priority on exercise and staying active as a family, our kids love running around outside playing. They all love playing sport and going for a bike ride. They do a lot of walking in their inner city neighbourhood and they have a lot of stamina to keep going.

The kids are totally accepting of my regular exercise routine. They love hearing about how I go with the latest fitness test or physical challenge. Baby Darcy learned to say 'push-up!' and jumped on my back to make it harder. I am pleased to be setting a good example for my children, my daughter in particular – as a lot of girls lose their enthusiasm for exercise as they progress through high school.

5 Easy-to-Implement Actions

1. Eat a variety of complex carbohydrates, lean proteins and healthy fats at every meal

2. Limit empty calories

3. Eat breakfast

4. Always carry healthy snacks

5. Reduce or eliminate pre-made packaged foods

Nurture from the Inside Out

Preparation and Consistency are Key

How to Begin and Stay on Track on YOUR Best Ever Body Journey

Working with many mums there are a few key mistakes that I see happen time and time again. The best education I can give you is to tell you what I have learned from others about what stops them from achieving their best ever body. Hopefully, with this information under your belt, you can go forth and really make a difference to your life and that of your family while discovering YOUR best ever body.

Top Five Mistakes

Mistake: Not planning

Whenever you make the decision to change something or do something new it's important to have a plan. Even more so now that you have a baby and are no longer a free agent – you do need to have routines in place. I'm not saying for a second that routines are fail-safe and we all know that with a baby the day you feel like you finally have a routine will be the day that they throw a curveball and completely change it. But, for you, your sanity and your wellbeing, you need to know that you have things planned into your day, and that some of those things are specifically there to nurture you and make you feel good.

You need to get good at scheduling your appointments into your day as rigidly as you do your child's doctor's appointment or swimming lesson. You wouldn't miss a swimming lesson to have coffee with a friend or get your hair done, and your training sessions or planned exercise should be the same. Even on the days that you don't feel like it, remember that energy creates energy and nine times out of ten you will feel better for honouring your commitment to yourself and getting moving.

Planning can relate to nutrition too. How many times have you decided you will ditch the sugar and junk foods and start eating healthily on Monday, only to get to the fridge on

How to love your body as much as your baby

Monday morning and discover you only have leftover takea-ways and chocolate in there. You're too tired or too busy to go to the shops so you grab whatever you can and figure you will start on Tuesday. Tuesday is a similar story and by the time Wednesday comes around, the weekend is already in sight and you figure you'll just start next week instead. With a baby, or more than one small child, preparation is essential.

Solution: Plan

Take some time for yourself to at first figure out what you are trying to get done. Are you starting to exercise again or want-ing to overhaul your diet? I challenge you to take half an hour when your baby is sleeping to sit down and really think about what you would like to put into your life that isn't there already. If you are coming out of that first six-week baby bubble this may be as simple as making sure you get dressed and out of the door every day by 10am. You might feel ready to go and find an exercise group so you will need to do some research and find a program that is suitable for you (don't forget to use my resource section on my website to help with that).

Mistake: Lack of commitment

Think back to before you had a baby – even back then commit-ting to exercise and healthy eating could be a challenge and you really only had you and perhaps your partner to worry about. How many times would you have the best intentions to get up and go to the gym before work, to run on your lunch break, or to stop off at the gym on the way home? And really, how easy was it to allow something to come into your life that prevented you from getting there, when it came down to it? Couldn't get out of bed, couldn't get out of the office, had to stay late...the list goes on. So now add to this equation a real reason to be tired. Experiencing broken sleep night after night is tough on anyone. Now add a second, very uncooperative little person who every morning you also have to account for, get ready and haul out the door, and you can soon see how daily exercise can be quickly thrown into the too hard basket. I truly believe that you just need to get started and it will get easier, that energy creates energy and lack of energy and movement does the exact opposite. The slower you get and the less commitment you make the easier it is to let it fall by the wayside, and we all know how hard it is to break the cycle of non-exercise. It takes a while before hauling yourself to your next training session becomes easy again.

Solution: Commit

One of the best ways to ensure you commit to something is to put your money where your mouth is. For most of us, if we are feeling financial pain knowing that if we don't follow through we are wasting money, then we do everything in our power to avoid feeling that pain and to get the most out of our investment. Unlike many investments, which may be managed by others and seemingly out of your control, your health and fitness is a direct representation of the effort you put in and the

How to love your body as much as your baby

commitment you maintain. So in essence, to make the decision to either work one-on-one with a specialised personal trainer, or to find a mum's group exercise class, is a really great way of making that commitment to yourself.

By working alongside other mothers you will immediately feel less alone and like someone else is going through exactly what you are. Someone else battled to get out of the door this morning and just by turning up you have both shown fantastic commitment to yourselves, and your children will benefit from that also. Should you choose not to join a structured exercise group or work with a PT, at the minimum you need to find someone who you can meet daily or a few people you meet on different days to do some exercise; a walk, swim or jog. BUT these people cannot be people that would easily cancel on you – you don't want to let their circumstances affect your level of commitment. Alternatively, you can create accountability by joining our online group and making yourself accountable there.

Mistake: Going it alone

How hard is it to motivate yourself to do something when there is no one to keep you accountable? We have a live-in *au pair* who is wonderful and always makes sure she cleans up after herself as she goes along. I am not someone who is particularly motivated to clean or tidy. You know those people who claim to like to clean? I am not one of them! I know that if there is a pile of washing up to be done, and there is only me who will see it if it's not done, I simply won't do it. But if I know that in the morning someone else will be faced with a sink full of dishes that they didn't create then I am much more likely to do them. I have an expectation of others and it's only right that I honour that expectation and do for them as I wish to be done for me, no matter how much I don't feel like it.

Solution: The power of a group

The power of a group is amazing. Knowing you have more than one person who has your best interests at heart is invaluable. Finding a group that has common interests and, in this case, has also made the change to leading a healthier more active lifestyle, can only have a positive effect on you. They say you should always surround yourself with positive people who share similar values and desires to you, and this is no exception. Find that group who will help to spur you on towards your goals and who will support you along the way.

Mistake: Thinking this has a timeframe

I speak to many people and witness firsthand the view that a new exercise regime or healthy eating plan is 'just for the next five weeks'. At the end of the five weeks these people simply go back to doing what they were doing before because their time is up; they've seen some results and now they don't have to do any more. They talk about a fool being someone who does the same thing every single day and expects to see change. What should we say then about someone who instigates and puts lots of energy into change, only sustains it for a short period of time, and then expects the change they've seen to be maintained, despite knowing full well that when they did the very same thing before nothing changed?

Solution: Commit to a lifestyle change

Although within my group training sessions we do both eight- and twelve-week challenges, I continually talk about the journey that you are on being a lifestyle change. You would not be part of the challenge for eight weeks and then just go back to doing the same level of exercise and making the same poor food choices as you were doing beforehand. I do see a few people who take this limited timeframe attitude. But the majority do the first challenge and take away their new thinking, new habits and education, teach their families what they now know and introduce new habits to their children and partners. With their whole team on board, the eight or twelve weeks almost just pass them by and their body continues to make changes due to them sustaining the healthy habits and commitment to exercise that they have invested in themselves.

One of the best examples is Sally. Sally came to me at the beginning of our winter challenge in June 2012. Over the course of these 12 weeks Sally lost over 10 kilos – she was looking fantastic and feeling great. We had a gap of about six weeks between the end of the winter challenge and the start of the summer challenge and it would have been easy for Sally to have stalled at this point, revert back to some of her old habits and slowly but surely begin to put the weight back on. Instead, she maintained what she was doing; she had made a commitment to her lifestyle change and the further along this journey she got, and the more results she saw within herself, the more she felt driven to continue. Consequently, Sally continued to lose weight in between challenges and then lost another eight kilos on the second challenge. Creating the right mindset for a lifestyle change, rather than going for a quick fix, is essential to your long-term results, your long-term health and fitness, and that of your family.

Mistake: Going too hard, too soon

When you make the decision to get in shape and get fit you always start off raring to go and really enthusiastic. I see many people who really jump in the deep end, especially with their exercise routine and the restrictions they decide to put on their food intake. Their high intensity, challenging and demanding training schedule is put into place and they decide they will get up at 6am every morning to go for their run or hit the gym. They completely overhaul their diet and create such extreme measures that they are almost inevitably setting themselves up for failure. A plan like this can be hard for anyone to hold down, let alone when you have a new little person in tow.

Solution: Know this is a journey

Whenever I talk to the mums I work with I talk to them about their journey. I stress that everybody's journey is different, and that is exactly what I would like to say to you. You need to figure out what you want to achieve in the long-term and then look at the step-by-step process that you need to embark upon to get there. By choosing to make little, doable and achievable changes every day you are slowly but surely overhauling your choices and your habits and creating a long-term lifestyle change. Resist the temptation to go at it all or nothing. You are already adjusting to so much as a mother that by overloading yourself and creating too much pressure or self-expectation it will be too easy to become disillusioned and to just give up if you should fail. I certainly believe that lots of little changes, made slowly over time, and that can be maintained, is a much better plan in the long-term.

Real Mums

Kylie, mum to Isla(15m)

When I was pregnant, like other mums-to-be, I imagined exactly how my maternity leave would look. I would go to Centennial Park every day, join Body Beyond Baby and be in the best shape of my life. My daughter was born in January 2012 and as a new mum I found that not everything went to plan. The best shape of my life was on the back burner and days rolled into weeks, weeks into months – before I knew it I had been planning for a year to get myself back on track. My daughter was one and I still didn't have a rhythm. She was in a great routine, was sleeping well and was a happy and (dare I say it) an easy baby. It was me who was missing something, because I was miserable!

Rock bottom hit when I received an email detailing my redundancy. I didn't understand, I NEEDED to return to work. I was ready and looking forward to it. Working would provide me with rhythm, routine, distance to miss my daughter, and would give me my confidence back – I was sure of it.

While I was digesting what had happened, I came up with a business idea – 'Mum Society' – so I drew up a business plan. I had target businesses and target guest speakers. I wanted to support other mums in the same or similar career situations that were also trying to have it all. But, in that moment, I lacked the confidence or clarity to take it any further than the planning stage.

How to love your body as much as your baby

A little time passed and I figured I had nothing to lose, so I set up a business Facebook page and, as fate would have it, Jen Dugard liked Mum Society and posted, 'What a fantastic mission – aligns very well with what we are about at Body Beyond Baby.' Jen was on my target list of businesses and would hopefully be my first guest speaker.

I danced around the house and was over the moon. I had admired Body Beyond Baby (admittedly from afar) and couldn't believe that I had my first Facebook like from a business with similar values. I arranged to meet with Jen as quickly as I could and, in one meeting, felt so inspired by her business approach and her passion that I signed up to Body Beyond Baby that afternoon. There was no pressure from Jen to sign up; she did explain to me that as someone who had embarked on a business venture I would need to make time for myself to ensure my success.

Joining Body Beyond Baby and making a commitment to myself is the best decision I have ever made. In eight short weeks, I feel better than I did long before I fell pregnant and fell victim to the 'relationship injection'. I feel not only empowered and restored to my former self, I am stronger and fitter than I was before I fell pregnant.

The power of the group commitment has changed my existence; connecting with other mums by sharing and celebrating our achievements has helped me to stay focused and determined to achieve my own goals. I spend a lot less time at home and in my PJ's and am most definitely a much better mum and wife for it. Physically, I have transformed and am

Preparation and Consistency are Key

really happy about how I feel (so is my husband). I have the energy I need to chase my daughter and also the clarity and determination that I lacked when starting with my business. My launch event was successful and I have to thank Jen and Body Beyond Baby for being involved and, more importantly, for restoring my confidence and providing me with the head-space I needed to make my business dream a reality.

Taking care of myself is now my priority as a business owner and, for me, is the most important part of being a mum. I am yet to reach my goal of my best body but I know for certain that it is in my future.

Danette, mum to Luella(2)

My change of life journey started when my daughter was about eight weeks old. My sister-in-law was exercising after having her daughter; she was looking fabulous and enjoying herself to boot. I had always been relatively fit and weight conscious, but when I fell pregnant with Lu I had gone through a number of IVF processes that left me well over my ideal weight and I was in a job that involved working with a very talented French chef, so you could say it was a recipe for disaster.

Lu came five weeks early so my planned relaxation never happened. I finished work on the Friday and she decided to come on the Monday. I did all the normal things – I joined a mothers group, we met in the park for coffee and cake...someone would always bake. I became friends with all the cafe owners as they would always see me walking the pram. They gave me a cake

How to love your body as much as your baby

to take home and share with my husband almost every day. Good grief, I was walking everywhere but nothing was going anywhere.

I started training regularly on a Tuesday morning. I loved seeing all the mums and what they had achieved, but I was unfit. What was even worse is that I didn't realise how unfit I was. Jen would lead me but still needed to push me, as I have to admit I was the worst complainer ever. How she did not kick me out is beyond me! My knees hurt therefore no burpee's for me...my back hurt so no prone hold for me, I thought. How could they hold a prone for over a minute? That was just crazy!

I trained and worked hard at getting my core back to where it should be, but sometimes I would get so frustrated at what I felt was the slowness of the process. But I had gotten stronger and fitter and was starting to look like the old me. I joined Jen's first challenge and decided to go cold turkey on sugar....yup, the whole family did. I still remember standing in the park telling Jen that I wanted to get fitter and feel amazing again! Doing the challenge gave me a clear objective to begin with, which was great. I do not own scales; I still don't but the first testing and measurements gave me a great starting mark and an idea of what needed to be changed. As soon as my mind-set changed and I challenged MYSELF, that is when it clicked for me.

The challenge finished just before Christmas and our family took a holiday up to Port Douglas for 10 days. Every day I was up at dawn and did a sand run or set up my own circuit session. Over the Christmas break I got stronger, fitter and leaner. I was inspired; I did this on my own with the tools that Jen had taught to me.

That January I went back to full-time work. I was petrified that my new-found love of fitness would suffer. I ran my diary like a well-oiled machine; planning sessions, learning to get out of bed by 5am most mornings to push myself. I learned to love running and set myself a challenge to do a running event in Centennial Park. Jen had set up a team to do it and it was great running with a huge contingent of females. I ran the whole event and I was so incredibly proud of myself.

But then my big love was found... I love training within a group and we signed up a team to complete an obstacle race.. It was dirty, it was messy, I got cuts and bruises and I loved it! This is how I was meant to train and have fun. My whole thinking changed – I needed to get stronger and I needed to get even fitter. I needed to start lifting weights. My running speed was at a good pace and my cardio was strong, but my upper body strength was not great. I stepped up my training with Jen and we introduced weights so I could be strong for challenges. I am relatively little and I was nervous that I would end up looking like a Romanian shot-putter, but weights have added a dimension that has slimmed down my arms and given me the tummy that I have always wanted! I look better now at 40 than I ever did in my 30s.

Every week is a challenge, organising my training around a busy husband (who is amazingly supportive), a job that I have to travel for and a two and a half year old. Training is a priority – it takes planning and a lot of early mornings. I absolutely

How to love your body as much as your baby

love it. I often get asked am I one of those people who just bounce out of bed to fit in my training, and I'm honest. No, my alarm goes off and I just get up and get ready. I'm awake by the time I drive out of our driveway.

My calendar up until Christmas is planned. It is pinned up above my desk so I can see the events that I am training for, and it gets me excited and motivated to be ready for those. To see the evolution in my training is amazing for me, but each little goal that I kick pushes me further.

5 Easy to Implement Actions:

1. Plan before you begin – write those goals down and put them somewhere you can see them regularly

2. Make a commitment – either make plans to meet someone in a certain place at a certain time or commit to group training sessions, a gym or personal trainer

3. Find a group to exercise with – make it fun and socialise at the same time

4. Make sustainable changes – writing little easy to reach goals each day can help things seem less challenging

5. Block out any pressure or noise from others – own your own journey and go at your own pace.

Preparation and Consistency are Key

Teach your Child Great Habits

How Educating Yourself will Benefit your Children

As a parent myself, and through my work with mothers and their children, I see how when mum makes the decision to really educate herself on healthy eating on a daily basis, and to making time for herself to exercise, that it filters through to the rest of the family. It is my belief that as mothers we have the huge responsibility of teaching our children how to eat. Simple as that may sound, I am sure there are many of you reading this who have been confused about what is healthy to eat, what the best choices are, how much and what type of exercise we should be doing blah blah blah... We have all heard it all before, but the fact is that as generations go by our children are moving less and less. The market becomes more saturated with video games and computers, we have the fear of not letting them roam the streets and so children aren't playing in that same physical way as they have done in the past. Add to this the growing amount of packaged and convenience foods laden with sugar and additives and no wonder we are facing the daunting thought that some of us will outlive our children, due to the huge increase in sedentary related diseases among our children.

Sugar and your Children

Is sugar really the devil everyone says it is? In my opinion, yes. How many of you, as grown women, are more addicted to sugar than anything else in your life? And not just sugar in typical sugar form – how many of you label bread as your 'thing'? And if you cut out one form of sugar, then how many of you then overload yourself on the 'healthy' forms of sugar i.e. fruit? Cut out the chocolate and consume a whole watermelon – sound familiar? And if sugar wasn't the enemy, if it was fat as we have been lead to believe for years and years, then why are we still getting fatter? Surely all of those low-fat and fat-free products we have been consuming should be making us slimmer? Have you checked the ingredients of most of those products? If it's low-fat then generally it's higher in sugar or some other kind of chemical sweetener. Then we pass our sugar addiction on to our children.

Have you seen what happens to your children after they consume sugar? The birthday parties where they gorge themselves on copious amounts of lollies and chocolates and cakes, soft drinks and popper juices? They run around like crazy, like animals needing to be let out of a cage, and then they crash, they come down. Just like you off alcohol – there are tears and upsets and tiredness. Their little bodies unravelling from the overstimulation and high they have just been through – the chemical reactions in their tiny bodies that cause them to ride the roller coast of high and then low and we allow this to happen. Because it's socially acceptable to do this to our children. Or because you don't feel like you can say no. No to something that you know will end up in tears but because everyone else is doing it and it's a 'one off' then its okay. I'd like to challenge you to really think about how much of a one off eating huge amounts of sugar is in your child's life. What does a typical day look like for them?

Here's an example of what I often find:

Breakfast – cereal; Weetbix, Nutrigrain or some other kind of out of a box, processed foods

Morning tea – sultanas, crackers, piece of fruit

Lunch – sandwich and a piece of fruit

Afternoon tea – sugary treat (because they've had no other sugar that day)

Dinner – pasta

Now in a typical day like this for the outset it doesn't look too bad right? But when you break it down to the sugar contained in every single meal or snack, and the way in which the body reacts to these foods, then they have been overloaded from morning till night. Going on mini roller-coaster rides all day long, and they are doing this day in day out.

It's time to break this cycle, and with the education you have given yourself you can overhaul your child's diet too. For those of you who have tiny babies and are yet to navigate the what to and when to feed your children, then you are the lucky ones – you can really make educated choices for your children based on your knowledge.

Busting the 'you just have to give it to them' Theory

I remember a little while ago chatting to a client about children's foods, what I give my children and what I say no to. I was telling her about my saying no to some chocolate that had been offered to my son (which I do regularly).She told me that if I continued to do that I would be the most hated mum at kindy – that if I put healthy foods into his lunch box then he wouldn't eat them. My answer – I don't care. I am not out to be liked, I am not out to conform, I am here to do what I believe is the best for my children and for me. A big part of that is ensuring that their little growing bodies are filled with the most nutritious, clean foods possible to help them grow and do everything they want to do and to set them up for the rest of their lives. Right from day one I have steered clear of processed foods, packaged food and sugary foods. My son did not have any of his birthday cake for the first three years of his life, did he care? He didn't know. A child who is just turning one, two or even three has absolutely no concept of missing out. It is us, as parents, as adults who put our own thoughts onto them. For a long time we had little, homemade, sugar free, mini muffins that would be pulled out at the same time as all the other kids were being given birthday cakes, cupcakes or any other treats we chose not to give to him. He didn't know the difference – he was eating what he had always known. I often see the look on other parents' faces when I refuse something on behalf of my children. My children are not missing out; I am making a decision which I believe is the right one for them.

There is a big difference in you, as an educated adult, making the decision to eat junk foods and sugary foods on occasion, and a child being given it to eat, who knows no better, cannot make a decision for themselves on what is the best choice and trusts you to do that for them.

My Story

I remember the first year that Marley was in kindy. He started in January at two and a half years old, and in April they were doing an Easter Egg Hunt. This was the first time I got a phone call from his teachers asking if he could have some chocolate. I remember standing in David Jones at the cash register completely taken by surprise (but grateful they had thought to call as they were aware of my views and wishes). I was told they were doing the Easter Egg Hunt and that they were tiny little

Easter eggs – until this time Marley had never had chocolate and whenever confronted by the shiny wrappers and colourful treats he would be more likely to be fascinated and play with them rather than want to eat them. To this day he sill calls Smarties 'crunchy beans' as they haven't played a big enough role in his life for him to know junk foods by their actual names. Having been put on the spot and really not knowing what to do, I admit I caved and said he could have one, almost immediately regretting my decision to succumb to allowing him to do something just because everyone else was. I needn't have worried. When I arrived to pick him up that afternoon his teacher said he hadn't had any chocolate anyway. Apparently when the teachers held up an egg to ask the children what was inside, all the other children had yelled 'chocolate', whereas Marley had said 'chicks'. Very rightly knowing that chicks came from eggs and oblivious to the fact that this very pretty shiny egg was actually a sugar filled chocolate egg. It was at that moment that his teacher made the decision to give him something else. He was given a few crackers to eat while the other children ate their chocolate eggs, which he was completely happy with (and so was I). His teacher had realised at that point that he wasn't missing out because he just wasn't aware, and I am glad she over road my moment of weakness and made the decision best for him at that time.

Marley is four now and clearly understands the difference between sometimes food and everyday foods. He knows that sugar doesn't help you to grow big and strong and that it doesn't keep you healthy. You can't keep it from them forever but you most certainly can keep it to exactly that, sometimes. And for us, as a family, sometimes doesn't mean every Wednesday after swimming and Friday on the way home from kindy. Sometimes is exactly that, there is no schedule and it doesn't happen 'just because'. 'Sometimes' in our house in generally a birthday party. At kindy, when another child brings in a birthday cake Marley will ask his teachers to 'call Mummy to see if he is allowed'. As parents we have now made the decision that he is allowed a very small piece of birthday cake at these times at kindy and also at actual birthday parties, but he is very aware that after that one piece there is no more.

For some of you this may be a very different way of thinking; 'What's wrong with a bit of sugar?' you ask. And why not just let him have it when the other kids do? I worked quite hard to get jelly and ice cream taken off the menu at kindy, and to me the fact that they listened to me is fantastic. If little bits of this information can filter through bit by bit to other people then we will be improving the health of generations to come. I know I don't want situations where my child is given junk food dictated to me by others –if I make the decision that my children are to eat sugar due to a particular occasion then I want to be the one making that decision. Not because it's on a menu every Monday and Wednesday – there's no sometimes in knowing something will happen every week.

The biggest thing for me, as a parent, is knowing that the decisions I make for my child shape their future. That they rely solely on myself and my husband to nurture them in the best possible way, they trust that we will do the best things for

191

them and whatever we choose to feed them in their early days will become what they know and what is normal for them. Children naturally want to run around, jump and play – they have so much energy and it is up to me to make sure they get that energy from the best possible sources. Clean, healthy, nutritious foods. And to most certainly not put my addictions or supposed need for crap food onto them and into their mouths.

I remember being out with a friend quite some time ago. Marley was about 18-months old and her son was approaching 12-months. The kids were running around and Marley kept returning for bits of his lunch from time to time. The mother of the child we were there with was eating chocolate, and she proceeded to follow her 12-month old around feeding him this chocolate. The child was clearly not interested in eating at that time and even less interested in the chocolate, but she continued to follow him around, breaking off bits of chocolate and pretty much making him eat it. This has never, ever made sense to me. Surely as a grown up you know that there is absolutely no nutritional value in chocolate, that it is laden with sugar and can really only be bad for your child. It still amazes me when I am out shopping and I see children of two or three years of age sitting in their pram eating donuts or drinking cans of soft drink! What has gotten into the minds of the people caring for them to think that it was a smart thing to do and a good choice for their child? What is wrong with an apple or a sandwich? And not a Vegemite sandwich on white bread – don't get me started on that one!

How to love your body as much as your baby

Tips for Removing Sugar from your Child's Diet

Don't believe they need it or are missing out – your children know what you teach them, they are smarter than you think and if, from an early age you explain the different values of foods and what it will do for their growing bodies, they will take that on board and base their own thoughts and choices around that.

Always have healthy alternatives with you – that you can offer instead at those times when other kids are eating sugary snacks. I remember a mother once saying she had bought cupcakes for all the children (under four-years old – I held my tongue) but I did politely turn down her offer and gave Marley his mini muffins, which he was completely happy with.

Limit your own sugar and junk food intake around them – or better still don't eat it at all. The best way to teach your children is to lead by example. If they see you eating a chocolate bar at 3pm every afternoon, they are going to think that is normal. If you don't want to pass on a bad habit, then you need to not let your children become exposed to it. Give it up yourself – it wouldn't be a bad thing.

Make your views known to others and stand strong – there have been countless times that other parents have (tried) to make me feel like my children are missing out because I have refused to feed them junk. I don't care and I stand strong in the decisions I make which I believe are best for my children.

Educate your children and explain to them why – children are really smart. They are like little sponges and they love to know the reason why to pretty much everything. Feed their brains as well as their bodies and explain to them why you are making these choices for them. Explain to them why sugar isn't good for them, talk to them about how it won't help them run around and grow big and strong, and as they get bigger and if you do chose to allow them to eat it at times, you can talk to them about how it makes them feel.

Navigating Birthday Parties

Belinda Kirkpatrick, has children who are a little older than mine and she lives by pretty much the same no sugar philosophies that I do. We are not naive enough to think that you can completely ban sugar from a child's life, and there is the fine line of knowing that you need to let out the reins now and again and that you don't want them to gorge themselves when they do have the option of eating sugary foods. She uses these tactics when navigating a kid's birthday party invite.

Make sure they have eaten before they go – a good breakfast and then if the party isn't for a few hours, top them up with a healthy and yummy smoothie before they go. Kids still have that inbuilt mechanism that prevents them from overeating and generally tells them to stop when they are full.

Let them eat what they want at the party– (knowing they started the day well and they are not arriving hungry).

If they are given a goodie bag to take home let them eat it in the car on the way home – but have the rule that once you are home the goodie bag is thrown out; no keeping it in the cupboard for another day.

Talk to them about how they feel later on – most kids will be able to recognise the fact that their tummy feels funny, they feel extra tired and just not so great.

Explain to them that it is the high amount of sugar in the foods that they have chosen to eat that has made them feel that way.

Trust you are doing the right thing.

Give them a Variety of Food

Children will go through phases of eating certain foods and then rejecting them the next week. Teach your children about what vegetables are; teach them their names and talk about how they will make them big and healthy and strong. Tell them about the different food groups on their plate and that they need to eat something from each part. Children take in so much information and want to learn – you may be surprised at how much they actually listen, learn from and then implement of their own accord later on, when given the chance.

And don't give up. It is documented that it can take a number of times for a child to accept a new food given to them so if at first you don't succeed try, try again. What they don't like today they may love tomorrow.

Eat with your Child

If at all possible make the time to sit down and eat with your child. Eat the same or very similar meals as them so that they can see you eating the same things, which will in turn encourage them to eat it too. I speak to many mums who say that they struggle to get their children to eat of an evening, and on further investigation we find that mum and dad are never sitting to eat with them at the table. Aim to make family meal times happen as much as possible and I am sure you will see an improvement in your child's eating behaviours.

Invite them to Cook with You

I admit I am not the worlds most enthusiastic or best cook but what I do like is to make healthy snacks. I find it fun and I also feel that this is where a lot of children end up consuming too much sugar and salt – through store bought, convenience foods. I've found quite a passion in creating fun and treat like snacks that my children look forward to, and also enjoy creating with me. From sugar free muffins and banana bread, to ice-blocks and mini mousse-like desserts. Because I am often experimenting with these things there is no right or wrong and it means they can have fun too.

Limit their TV Time and Encourage them to Move

Technology is taking over our world and it still amazes me that my two-year old daughter can unlock my iPad, find her favourite games and could occupy herself for hours on end – if I let her. TV is the other big culprit in encouraging our children to be more sedentary. Where, when we were children, we would have gone out to play or occupied ourselves in some other way, young children often seem to want to take the easy option and sit in front of the box.

It is your job to be the parent; lay the ground rules and know what is best for them. Now that you will also be set in your exercise routine, you will be leading by example. My children know that mummy and daddy go to the gym, they know that we do our exercise because its good for us and they know that they get to go to the park and run around because it's good for them and keeps them healthy, fit and strong.

As children get older it can be more challenging but if you lay the foundations from the start it is much easier to encourage the upkeep of good habits rather than to reduce bad habits and implement new ones.

Real Mums

Kerry, mum to Avani (4) and Danan (2)

I totally concur with Jen's philosophy on food for kids! I think it's fair to say that my kids don't eat like most other kids. Their first food was soft boiled egg yolk mixed with cod liver oil and for my son I also added raw organic and grass-fed liver grated in with it! They moved onto avocado and bananas and vegetables but neither of them ate grains until about 11-months and even then, it was gluten free. They were both breastfed until around 13-months.

I followed a diet based on traditional societies as documented by the research of a dentist, Weston A Price. I took their nutrition extremely seriously and even now I see myself as succeeding or failing as a mother on a daily basis, dependent on what they have eaten! The diet basically follows a wholefood philosophy including organic vegetables, fruits, grass-fed meats, raw milk, bone broths, eggs, nuts and seeds. Both of my kids thrived and I somehow managed to avoid, as much as I possibly could, the things I consider non-foods; things in packets with numbers as ingredients, trans fats, soy, sugar...the list goes on and on! I read ingredient lists and am horrified that manufacturers can expect

How to love your body as much as your baby

people to eat some products, but people and, more scarily, kids do!!

My philosophy is that if I read an ingredient that I am unable to identify, I won't buy it. If there are certain numbers in the ingredients, I won't buy it (look out for 6's and 2's). If it contains sugar, soy, corn or any weird oil as an ingredient, I won't buy it. My kids eat fresh, real food, cooked in a non Teflon pan, and they have never eaten food prepared by me from a microwave. My daughter didn't know what the confectionary aisle was, and when we did venture down it once or twice, I told her the pretty packets were decorations and she bought it until she was nearly four!

So after saying all this and rating myself according to diet, imagine my dismay when at 10-months of age, my son developed a skin rash that I was told by doctors was eczema. When I think back, I realise that it appeared when we were staying at a holiday house that had a bit of a musty smell and seemed very dusty but I will probably never know if that triggered the rash.

The year following was the most difficult of my life. I was determined to find the source of the problem, and I was more determined to heal my son in a natural, safe and effective way. I have seen GPs, Paediatricians, dermatologists, herbalists, a Chinese doctor, naturopaths, and doctors who test EVERYTHING like blood, urine, hair and even poo. For over a year I slept (or rather didn't sleep) with my son to stop him scratching himself to bleeding. I bought allergy clothing, I covered him in natural fabrics so he couldn't scratch himself. I tried every type of topical treatment (even cortisone once, against my better judgment – it felt so wrong and I never did it again).I had a whole house water filter system fitted to my home and I tried every diet that sounded sensible!!

Finally I stumbled across the GAPS diet, written by a neurosurgeon to treat autism and Asperger's (she mentions that kids with these conditions often have eczema too). She is finding success with many conditions including autoimmune disorders. IT WORKS! We are still a work in progress but my son's skin is mostly clear and soft. If we go off the diet and one (or more) of the avoidance foods slips through, his skin flares the next day. The funny thing is that the diet is almost identical to the one I started them both on. The only difference is that I overlooked the fermented foods, which are a natural probiotic and great for the flora in the gut.

Following this diet has taught me that our gut flora is crucial to our health throughout life and can assist in avoiding many of the abundance of 'new' diseases we are suffering from in our society. The number one enemy, as far as I am concerned, is sugar. We are simply not supposed to eat as much as we do and people who say, 'But it's just a bit of birthday cake, what's the big deal?' should think about what else goes in on a daily basis. Sugar is in EVERYTHING. It is virtually impossible to avoid but for the sake of my kids' bodies and brains, I will do everything I can to allow them to enjoy a fun and carefree childhood without poisoning them at every opportunity.

My daughter is now attending preschool two days a week, which is the first time she has left my care in her life. I have requested a gluten and sugar free diet for her but because of this she misses out on every kids' birthday cake (quite frequently apparently!), so the teacher asked that I bring something to freeze for her to have while the other kids eat cake so she doesn't feel left out. I nearly relented and changed my mind so that my kid isn't the weird, left out one, but I didn't. She'll just have to get used to it. Hopefully one day she'll thank me because it's for the sake of her health.

I truly believe that one day in the foreseeable future, sugar will be seen as the evil that tobacco turned out to be. It's making us sick and it's killing us slowly. My kids don't miss out on anything. I make choc chip cookies, chocolate cakes, banana cakes etc. with grain and sugar free recipes. They eat chocolate (the real antioxidant type), they eat ice cream (made from cashew nuts and liquorice root) and they have milk-shakes (whey protein from organic pasture fed cows).I don't want them to feel like they are missing out because they're not; I just know there is a better alternative. I made my daughter a strawberry cake and my son a blueberry cake for their birthdays, sweetened with honey. They were great! I had people who eat 'normal' food telling me they were the best cakes they had ever eaten. Makes me wonder why if it can be done, why it isn't done more?

My kids will one day go out into the big wide world as I did and go nuts on everything they think they want to eat. I just hope that I can teach them well enough that they will get through that stage quickly and unscathed and come back to a world of health and vitality!!

Sharon, mum to Maddie (4)

As a parent, one of the responsibilities that I struggle with most, is food. In particular, what to feed my daughter, and how best to get her, the world's greatest food critic at the ripe old age of four, to eat the food I prepare. I struggle with the ever present challenge of how to educate her to make healthy food choices.

From my daughter's perspective healthy food is never going to have the appeal of junk food. Broccoli is never going to look as cool as "Dora the Explorer" yoghurt and raw almonds are never going to look as tasty as "Natural Confectionary" lollies. Marketing and clever packaging cause adults to reach for the unhealthy option, what hope does my four year old daughter have?

One technique I have devised is to create a game around making healthy choices. There is nothing more exciting for my daughter than a game that she can play, especially if it is a game that she can play with me. Our newest game is called "what foods make you strong?". We hit the supermarket and the question to be answered is "is this a food that will make you strong?". My daughter understands what it means to be strong, in the sense that, she can run faster or jump higher. She knows that to do this, she needs to eat food that will make her strong. She wants to be taller and read books and again we talk about the 'strong foods' that will help her achieve her simple little goals.

We play the game while we do the supermarket shop. I point to the display of tomatoes "Strong or no?" and she answers "strong Mummy". I point to the tins of tuna "Strong or no?" and she answers "Strong Mummy". We stroll through the supermarket aisles pointing and talking. Whenever we hit the 'sugar' aisle, it is a series of giggles over how many "not strong" foods there are. The game hasn't taken away my daughter's desire for junk food but it has started to educate her on making healthy choices. I have seen her choose fruit or veggie sticks over sugary or high fat foods. I have seen her request water or milk over a soft drink.

My daughter has started asking me for something to eat with the question of "will this sandwich/fruit/vegetables make me strong?". I love that she is thinking about what she is eating, and how in a very simplistic way considering what affect the food will have on her. I see the pride in her little face when she finishes her dinner and declares that she is stronger!

5 Easy to Implement Actions

1. Always have sugar free snacks on hand

2. Plan one or two occasions a week to cook with your child – try some sugar free muffins or other healthy snacks

3. For as long as they don't understand don't give them sugar, and when they are old enough to ask, talk to them and educate them about what helps them grow big and strong and what doesn't

4. Take your children with you when you exercise so it becomes part of their routine

5. Limit TV time and aim to have activity time instead

Teach your Child Great Habits

Time to Take Action

This is the section where you get to write your own program, where you get to become accountable and really start to work toward YOUR best ever body.

I'd like you to buy yourself a new notebook. A nice one, one that will be dedicated to you and will track your journey to YOUR best ever body.

Take some time out, find a time when your bub is sleeping or, even better, escape the house for a little while you can and start this journey by creating some you time.

What is YOUR Best Ever Body?

On the first page of your book I would like you to do the following:

- Describe YOUR best ever body
- What does it look like?
- What do you see in the mirror?
- How do you feel on the inside?
- What can your body do?
- What do people say about you?
- How do you feel emotionally?
- How do you feel mentally?
- What are your energy levels like?

Remember to talk as if you are already there, you can feel it, you are experiencing it.

Is there a picture of yourself from another time in your life that you would like to aim for? Is there a picture of someone else you would like to aim for? Stick this in your book.

Where Are You Right Now?

Take a photograph:

- Wear something tight (only you ever have to see these pictures), maybe take one in jeans and a tight singlet too in case you do want to show other people later
- Stick this picture in your book

How to love your body as much as your baby

AND Take your baseline measurements

- Choose how you will record where you are right now, use scales AND measurements or go get your skin folds or body composition scan done – write them done or stick your results into your book

Find out where you on your rebuild from the inside out journey:

- Check for abdominal separation. Do you have it? Write down your findings.
- Can you activate your pelvic floor or have you seen a women's health physio and had it checked? Write down your findings
- Can you activate your transverse abdominus effectively without oblique activation either through your own experimentation or through a visit to your women's health physio? Write down your findings

Perform some basic fitness testing which takes into account where you are on your rebuild journey:

- For example: How many push-ups can you do (if not due to pelvic floor or weakness or abdominal separation write this down)
- Time yourself running a certain distance (if you are able to run at this time)

Teach your Child Great Habits

To Change You Must Take Action

Do you need to book an assessment appointment with a physio?

If yes, write down your intention and then your appointment time and date

- What will you commit to in terms of exercise this week?
- How many days will you do your rebuilding exercises?
- How many walks will you do?
- How many resistance exercise sessions will you do?
- Write down answers to all of the above

Don't be afraid to start small – you can decide and alter this from week to week. You need to make it achievable so if it's one walk, one resistance session and rebuilding exercises every other day then that's a great place for you to start.

You can then raise the bar as you go.

What will you change within your diet this week?

Write down three things you will change.

I'd like you to visit what you have written down on a daily basis to begin with.

Tick off when you have achieved what you have set out to do for that day/week.

On a Sunday you will review your exercise and nutrition goals from the week before and refine them for the week ahead until you are mentally and physically in a place where you can maintain a balanced weekly routine of rebuilding, cardio, resistance and make changes to your diet as you go.

Some weeks you will do more, some weeks you may do less.

Now if you haven't done it already, come join us on Facebook, share your goals, make yourself accountable, make use of the community and encouragement that is there to help you on your way and keep me posted as to how you are going.

Remember, I am here for you to ask questions too so anytime you are unsure, would like to know more about something or need a little pep talk hop online and ask away.

I look forward to seeing you there!

Jen

References

Happy Mummy, Happy Baby

beyondblue fact sheet number 8

Jorm AF, Christensen H, Griffiths KM, Korten AE, Rodgers B. *Help for depression: What works (and what doesn't).* Centre for Mental Health Research: Canberra, 2001.

Rebuild from the Inside out

Ashton-Miller J, Delancey J, (2001) The functional anatomy of the female pelvic floor and stress continence control system. *Scandinavian Journal of urology and Nephrology supplement* 207.

Boissonnault, J, Blaschak, M (1988). Incidence of diastasis recti abdominis during childbearing year. *Physical Therapy* 68, 7.

DeLancey, J, (2002) Fascial and muscular abnormalities in women with urethral hypermobility and anterior vaginal wall prolapse. *American Journal of Obstetrics and Gynaecology* 187 (1): 93-98

Dietz H, Benneett, M, (2003) The effect of childbirth on pelvic organ mobility. *Obstetrics and Gynaecology* 102(2): 223-228.

How to love your body as much as your baby

Dietz H, Steensma (2006) the role of childbirth in the aetiology of recrocele. *British Journal of Obstetrics and Gynaecology* 113: 264-267.

Gutke A, Ostgaard, H Oberg, B (2008)Predicting persistent pregnancy related low back pain. *Spine* 33: E386-E393.

Hodges P, Richardson C, (1999) Altered trunk muscle recruitment in people with low back pain and upper limb movement at different speeds. *Archives of Physical Medicine and Rehabilitation.* 80: 1005.

Hodges P, Sapsford, R, Pengel L (2007). Postural and respiratory functions of the pelvic floor muscles. *Neurology and Urodynamics* 26: 362.

Lee D, Lee L, McLaughlin L (2008) Stability, continence and breathing: The role of fascia following pregnancy and delivery. *Journal of bodywork and movement therapies* 12: 333-348.

Pool-Goudzwaard A, Slieker M, Muider P, Snijders C, Stoeckart R (2005) Relations between pregnancy related low back pain, pelvic floor activity and pelvic floor dysfunction International *Urogynecology Journal* 16: 468-474

Smith M, Russell A, Hodges P, (2006a) Disorders of breathing and continence have a stronger association with back pain than obesity and physical activity. *Australian Journal of Physiotherapy* 52: 11.

Smith M, Coppieters M, Hodges P, (2008) Is balance different in women with and without stressurinary incontinence? *Neurourology and Urodynamics* 27: 71-78.

Smith M, Coppieters M Hodges P (2007b) Postural response of the pelvic floor and abdominal muscles in women with and without incontinence. *Neurourology and Urodynamics* 26(3): 377-388.

Thompson J, O'Sullivan P, Briffa N (2006) Altered muscle activation patterns in symptomatic women during pelvic floor muscle contraction and valsalva manoeuvre. *Neurourology and Urodynamics* 10: 268-274.

Wilson P, Herbison P, Glazener C, McGee M, MacArthur C (2002) Obstetric practice and urinary incontinence 5-7 years after delivery. ICS proceedings *Neurology and Urodynamics.* 21(4) 284-300.

Wu W, Meijer O, Uegaki K (2004) Pregnancy related pelvic girdle pain (PPP) I: Terminology, clinical presentation and prevalence. *European Spine* 13(7): 575-581.

Hodges P, Sapsford, R, Pengel L (2007). Postural and respiratory functions of the pelvic floor muscles. *Neurology and Urodynamics* 26: 362

How to love your body as much as your baby

Building the fancy house

Physiological adaptations to low-volume, high-intensity interval training in health and disease. Martin J Gibala,1 Jonathan P Little,2 Maureen J MacDonald,1 and John A Hawley3

Considerable evidence currently exists to support a role for low-volume HIT as a potent and time-efficient training method for improving your health. *http://www.ncbi.nlm.nih.gov/pmc/articles/PMC3381816/*

Nurture from the inside out

List of where sugar hides; Six Pack Chick, *Change your Mind, Transform your Body,* Brigdet Hunt. ecademy press, 2012

I hope you enjoyed reading my book - I'd love to answer your questions, continue the conversation and meet you in our community.

- Come and say hello on Facebook @Jen Dugard or Body Beyond Baby
- Follow me on Twitter @JenDugard
- Look at my pretty pictures on Instagram @JenDugard
- Check out my website and blog - *www.jendugard.com*
- Send me an email jen@jendugard.com

Body Beyond Baby
First published in Australia in 2013
www.jendugard.com

National Library of Australia Cataloguing-in-Publications entry

Author: Jen Dugard
Title: How to Love Your Body as Much as Your Baby
Illustrations © Natalie Jasper 2013
Photography © Mikey Pozarik 2013
Edited by Green Olive Press
Cover design by Pam Partridge
Internal design by Marley Berger
Produced by OpenBook Creative

ISBN: 9780987523006 (paperback)

Subjects: Mothers — Health and hygiene.
         Motherhood — Health aspects.
         Body image.
         Physical fitness for women.
         Motherhood in popular culture.

Dewey Number: 613.7045

All the information, exercises, ideas and examples contained within this publication are of the nature of general comments only, and not in any way recommended as individual advice. The intent is to offer a variety of information based on the current exercise guidelines and industry practice to provide a wider range of choices now and in the future, recognizing that we all have widely diverse circumstances. Should any reader choose to make use of information contained herein without obtaining specific advice for their circumstances, this is their decision, and the contributors, author and publishers do not assume any responsibilities whatsoever under any conditions or circumstances. It is recommended that the reader obtain their own independent advice.

www.ingramcontent.com/pod-product-compliance
Lightning Source LLC
Chambersburg PA
CBHW072119020426
42334CB00018B/1650